T0277073

*Alzheimer*

# Alzheimer

## The Life of a Physician and the Career of a Disease

KONRAD MAURER & ULRIKE MAURER

*Translated by Neil Levi, with Alistair Burns*

Columbia University Press
New York

Columbia University Press
*Publishers Since 1893*
New York   Chichester, West Sussex
Copyright © 1998 Piper Verlag GmbH, München
Translation copyright © 2003 Columbia University Press

Library of Congress Cataloging-in-Publication Data
Maurer, Konrad, 1943–
[Alzheimer—das Leben eines Arztes und die Karriere einer Krankheit, English]
Alzheimer : the life of a physician and the career of a disease / Konrad Maurer and
Ulrike Maurer.
p.   cm.
Includes bibliographical references and index.
ISBN 978-0-231-11896-5 (cloth : alk. paper)
1. Alzheimer, Alois  2. Neurologists—Germany—Biography
3. Psychiatrists—Germany—Biography  4. Alzheimer's disease—Research—History
I. Maurer, Ulrike, 1942–  II. Title.

RC339.52.A45 M3813 2003
616.8'092—dc21
[B]   2002041014

Columbia University Press books are printed on permanent and
durable acid-free paper.

*Designed by Chang Jae Lee*

Printed in the United States of America

*To Robert N. Postlethwait, Jochen Becker,*
*and the five granddaughters and grandson of Alois Alzheimer*

# Contents

# Preface

The whole world speaks of Alzheimer's, the incurable disease that afflicts so many older people. Yet Alois Alzheimer, after whom the disease is named, remains largely unknown.

Alzheimer was an obsessed doctor and scientist. By day he calmly examined his patients and cared for them tenderly; deep into the night he sat at his microscope and studied slides of the brain that he had prepared himself. His contemporaries called him "the psychiatrist with the microscope" because he was convinced that mental illnesses were diseases of the brain, in stark contrast to the then-burgeoning approach of psychoanalysis, which traced psychological problems to traumatic childhood experiences. An unavoidable clash between the two sides took place at a conference in 1906. Alzheimer stood there as his contribution on the case of Auguste D. met with no interest; the minutes of the proceedings called it "inappropriate for a brief report."

Yet just a few years later presenile dementia, from which only a few people suffered at that time, began to receive greater attention. *Presenile dementia*, or *Alzheimer's disease*, quickly emerged as one of the most frequently used disease names in the history of medicine. However, Alois Alzheimer did not live to see these events: He died in 1915 at age 51.

Fifty years later, life expectancy in the industrialized world had doubled. Alzheimer's disease claimed its first prominent victims: The world was shaken when actress Rita Hayworth was diagnosed with Alzheimer's. Hope continued that it would remain, as Alzheimer himself described it, a "peculiar disease." But when Ronald Reagan said farewell to his compatriots in a 1994 letter stating that he had Alzheimer's, people around the world finally became aware of the seriousness of the disease. Today, 30 to 40 million people are afflicted with this illness worldwide.

In private life Alois Alzheimer was a loving, imaginative, and often lively man who never forgot his roots in the German region of Franconian Spessart. Insight into his life and works was made possible only through many personal conversations with his descendants and by means of a family tree produced for this book. The authors especially want to thank

Alzheimer's granddaughters, Hildegard Koeppen, Ilse Lieblein, Barbara Lippert, and Karin Weiss; and his grandson, Dr. Rupert Finsterwalder. With their help, the museum at the Marktbreit birthplace of their grandfather was established.

We sincerely thank Andrea Schultheis for her inexhaustible and creative commitment to transcribing the text and Dr. Hubert Hess for his informed and critical revision of the book.

Thanks must go to Markus Dockhorn and Dr. Klaus Stadler of Piper Verlag and to Linda Strehl for their assistance with the manuscript. Finally, thanks also to Neil Levi and Alistair Burns.

*Ulrike and Konrad Maurer*

Frankfurt, July 1998

*Alzheimer*

# 1. *The Auguste D. File*

*November 26, 1901*

"What is your name?"[1]

   "Auguste."

   "Family name?"

   "Auguste."

   "What is your husband's name?"

   "I believe Auguste."

   "Your husband?"

   "Oh, my husband . . ."

   "Are you married?"

   "To Auguste."

   "Mrs. D.?"

   "Yes, to Auguste D."

   "How long have you been here?"

   "Three weeks."

   "What do I have in my hand?"

   "A cigar."

   "Right. And what is that?"

   "A pencil."

   "Thank you. And that?"

   "A steel nib pen."

   "Right again. What is that, Mrs. D.?"

   "Your purse, doctor."

   "Yes. Right. And that?"

   "A book."

   "And what is lying next to my notebook?"

   "A bunch of keys."

   "What does it consist of?"

FIGURE 1.1 *Auguste D., the first patient with Alzheimer's Disease*

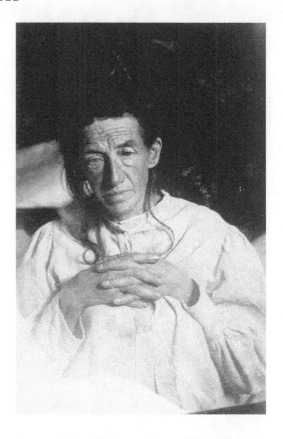

"Individual keys."

Dr. Alzheimer, senior physician at the Asylum for the Insane and Epileptic in Frankfurt am Main, just wanted to get an overview of the new admittees from the previous day. At first he only glanced at this file, but he simply could not put it down again: Auguste D., wife of a railroad clerk, born May 16, 1850. His assistant, Dr. Nitsche, had examined the patient the day before, between 10 and 11 o'clock. But Dr. Alzheimer sensed that there was something special about Auguste D. He decided to examine her himself. He did not yet know, on that gloomy November day, that he was making the most momentous decision of his life.

At midday Auguste D. had cauliflower and pork for lunch.

"What are you eating?"

"Spinach!"

She chewed the meat.

"What are you eating now?"

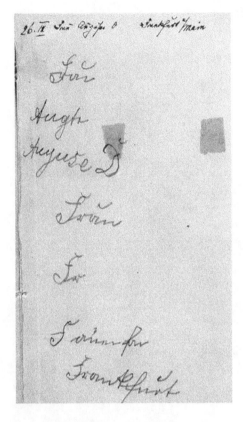

FIGURE 1.2 *A sample of Auguste D.'s handwriting*

"First I eat the potatoes and then the horseradish."

Dr. Alzheimer showed her several objects. After a short time she no longer knew what she had been shown. In between she spoke repeatedly of "twins."

"Write 'Mrs. Auguste D.'"

She wrote "Mrs.," but she forgot the rest. She could write her full name if she was told each individual word. Instead of "Auguste," however, she wrote "Auguse."

She had trouble putting sentences together and showed signs of verbal perseveration.

Dr. Alzheimer was satisfied with the result of his first examination. He put her name and the date next to the sample of Auguste D.'s writing. He had never seen a patient forget her own name while writing. He described her behavior as an "amnesic writing disorder" and decided to continue his examination of Auguste D.

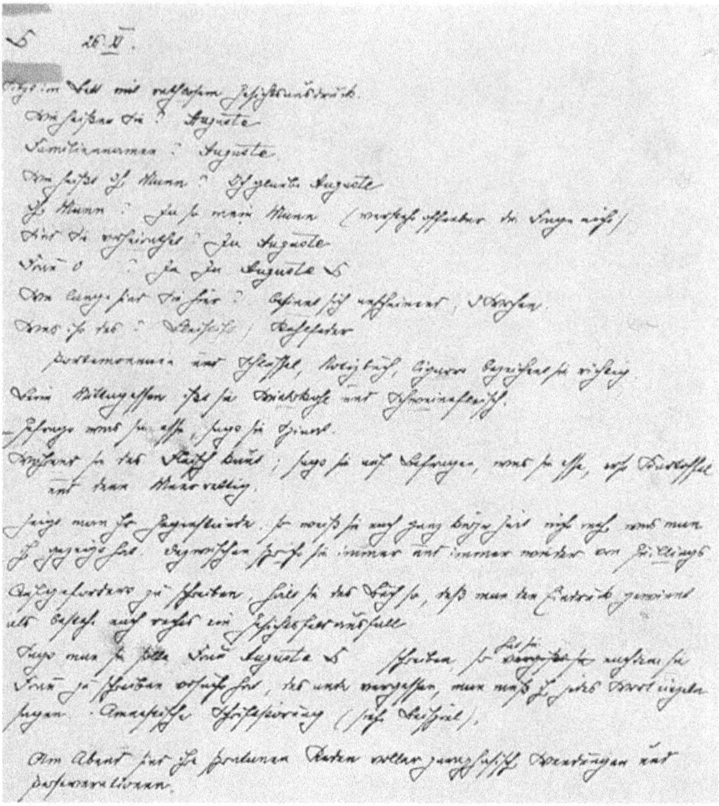

FIGURE 1.3 *Alzheimer's admission findings from November 26, 1901*

## November 28, 1901

Auguste D. was constantly fearful and at a loss. She said, over and over, "I won't let myself be cut," acted as if she were blind, walked about, groped the faces of other patients, and was struck by them in return. When asked what she was doing, she said, "I have to tidy up."

## November 29, 1901

She was placed in an isolation room, where she behaved quite calmly. When Alzheimer came in, she was again lying helplessly in bed.

"How are you?"

THE AUGUSTE D. FILE    5

"It all comes to the same thing. So who carried me here?"

"Where are you?"

"At the moment; I have temporarily, as said, I don't have means. One has to just—I don't know myself—I don't know at all—oh, goodness gracious, what is it all?"

"What is your name?"

"Mrs. D. Auguste!"

"When were you born?"

"Eighteen hundred and . . ."

"In which year were you born?"

"This year, no, past year."

"When were you born?"

"Eighteen hundred—I don't know."

"What did I ask you?"

"Oh, D. Auguste . . ."

"Do you have children?"

"Yes, a daughter."

"What is her name?"

"Thekla!"

"How old is she?"

"She is married in Berlin, Mrs. Wilke."

"Where does she live?"

"We live in Cassel!"

"Where does your daughter live?"

"Waldemarstrasse—no, different . . ."

"What is your husband's name?"

"I don't know . . ."

"What name does your husband have?"

"My husband isn't here right now."

"What is your husband's name?"

She answered all at once, quickly and as if she were waking up.

"August Wilhelm Karl; I don't know if I can state it just like that."

"What is your husband?"

"Clerk—I'm so mixed up—so mixed up—I can't."

"How long have you been here?"

"Two days probably . . ."

"Where are you?"

"That is probably Wilhelmshöhe."

"Where is your apartment?"

"Well, Frankfurt . . ."

"On which street?"

"Not Waldemarstrasse, so another, wait a moment; I am so very, so very . . ."

"Are you ill?"

"More downward, along the spine . . ."

"Do you know me?"

"I believe you have already treated me twice; no, excuse me, I can't so . . ."

"What year are we living in?"

"Eighteen hundred . . ."

"Which month?"

"Second month."

"What are the names of the months?"

Auguste D. rapidly recited the names of the months correctly.

"Which month is it now?"

"The eleventh."

"What is the eleventh month called?"

"So, the last—no, not the last . . ."

"Which?"

"I don't know so . . ."

"What color is snow?"

"White."

"Soot?"

"Black."

"The sky?"

"Blue."

"Grass?"

"Green."

"How many fingers do you have?"

"Five."

"Eyes?"

"Two."

"Legs?"

"Two."

"How many pfennigs make a mark?"

"A hundred."

"What does an egg cost?"

"Six or eight."

"Six or eight what?"

"Yes."

"Six or eight marks?"

"Yes, marks."

Dr. Alzheimer asked again about everyday things and asked her to do some arithmetic.

"What does a pound of meat cost?"

"Seventy."

"Seventy what?"

"I don't know . . ."

"A roll?"

"3 pfennigs."

"$2 \times 3$?"

"6."

"$9 \times 7$?"

"63."

"$12 \times 19$?"

"27."

"$6 \times 8$?"

"48."

"$4 \times 12$?"

"48."

"If you buy six eggs at seven pfennigs each, what does that make?"

"Poaching."

"Which street do you live in?"

"I can't tell you that, I just have to wait a moment."

"What did I ask you?"

"So, that is Frankfurt."

"On which street do you live?"

"I can't tell you that, Waldemarstrasse—not, no."

"When did you get married?"

"I don't know that at the moment; indeed, the woman lives on the same corridor."

"Which woman?"

"The woman, where we live." Then she called loudly, "Mrs. Hensler, Mrs. Hensler, Mrs. Hensler. . . . She lives down here a level."

Again Alzheimer showed Auguste D. objects and had her read and write. She correctly named keys, a pencil, and a book.

"What have I shown you?"

"I don't know. . . . I don't know . . . so nervous, so nervous."

Dr. Alzheimer held up three fingers. "How many fingers am I holding up?"

"Three."

"Are you still nervous?"

"Yes."

"How many fingers did I show you?"

"Well, it's Frankfurt."

Dr. Alzheimer set out before Auguste D. a series of objects that she was meant to recognize by touch, with her eyes closed. Toothbrush, bread, roll, spoon, brush, glass, knife, fork, plate, purse, a mark piece, a cigar, and a key; she named them quickly and without difficulty. She described a metal cup as a milk pourer with a teaspoon. When she opened her eyes she said immediately, "A cup."

Her writing was the same as in previous days. Instead of "Mrs. Auguste D." she wrote "Mrs."; the rest she had forgotten and had to be told over and over again. As she wrote she said repeatedly, "I have, so to speak, lost myself."

In her reading she skipped between lines; some lines she read five times over. She appeared not to understand what she read; she stressed the words in unusual ways. Suddenly she spontaneously said the name "Quilling."

"Of course you know the Quillings?" During the rest of the examination she dwelled on the name "Quilling."

Dr. Alzheimer also performed a thorough physical examination. Apart from being underweight, she was physically normal. The apex beat was not palpable, the heart was not enlarged, and the pulmonic second sound was not audible.

At the center of his examination were the neurologic findings. The pupils reacted normally to incident light. The tongue, when stuck straight out, barely quivered but was extremely dry because of inadequate fluid intake. She wore dentures. She showed no disturbances in articulation.

However, Auguste D. often interrupted herself while pronouncing words, as if she were at a loss or undecided as to whether what she was saying was correct.

During the examination she carried out all requests with rapid comprehension. She did not show signs of nervousness but did say suddenly, "A child just called! Is it there?"

"Do you often hear someone calling?"

"But you know Mrs. Quilling, of course!"

As she was to be taken from the isolation room to her bed she got worked up, screamed loudly, struggled, showed great fear, and called repeatedly, "I will not be cut! I will not let myself be cut!"

## *November 30, 1901*

Auguste D. often went into the main room, grabbed the faces of the other patients, and hit them. Because no one knew why she did this, she was isolated. Undeterred, Dr. Alzheimer continued his investigation.

"I don't feel like it and I don't have time."

"For what?"

"I would very much like to ask myself that."

"How are you?"

"It was quite good the last few days."

"Where are you?"

"Here and everywhere—here and now—you mustn't take offense."

"Where are you?"

"We will still live there."

"Where is your bed?"

"Where should it be?"

"How did you sleep last night?"

"Quite well."

"Where is your husband?"

"At the office; clerk, first class . . ."

"How old are you?"

"Fifty-seven years."

"Where do you live?"

"Waldemarstrasse . . ."

"Have you already eaten something today?"

"Yes, soup and various things."

"What are you doing now?"

"Yes, cleaning or something like that."

"Why haven't you gotten dressed?"

"I had things to do."

"How long have you been here?"

"You had written it down—fifty-seven."

"Fifty-seven what?"

She remains silent.

Auguste D. continued to behave strangely. She soon sent Alzheimer out of the room: "Please, you have no business being here."

Then she greeted him again as if he were a guest: "Do you want to take a seat? It's just that I still haven't had any time."

Later she pushed him out of the isolation room again and cried out loudly, like a child. Then she fell into a delirium in which she carried around her bedding, folded together the sheets and blanket, and sometimes shoved everything under the bed. She perspired from fear and repeatedly called "Karl" and "Thekla," the names of her husband and daughter.

Alzheimer asked her again, "What is your husband's name?"

"August!"

"Where are you?"

"At home." Sometimes she also said, "In the hospital."

Alzheimer had the impression that she no longer simply misunderstood but also was unable to do things. He instructed her, "Knit."

Auguste D. pulled all the needles out of her knitting and began to remove stitches from the middle. Alzheimer asked her what kind of furniture the commode was.

"That is my commode, please close the lid!"

## Early December 1901

As on the previous day, Auguste D. sat in bed helplessly, with a fearful expression. When Alzheimer entered the room she regarded him suspiciously. During the conversation she was tearful and reflected on her answers for a long time.

"You do not seem happy to see me at all," she said.

"Why?"

"I don't know. We didn't have debts or anything like that. I'm just nervous, you can't take offense at that."

"What is your name?"

"Mrs. Auguste D."

"What are you?"

"Mrs. Auguste D."

"How old are you?"

"Fifty-one."

"Where do you live?"

"Birthday? In Cassel."

"Where do you live?"

"Of course, you have already been to our house. Oh, I was only so nervous, please, please."

"Where do you live?"

"Mörfelder Landstrasse."

"Right! What year is it now?"

"One moment, I'm so nervous. So, how old am I? Fifty-one."

"What month is it?"

"The sixth—no—so, fifty-one. Yes, doctor, what have I done then, just tell me."

"What is today's date?"

"Fifty-one—no, I—am a bit nervous. Is that so bad, doctor? I don't know about anything."

"What day of the week is it today?"

"Sixty-five. Oh God, I used to be much better at sums."

"How long have you already been here?"

"Fifty-one."

"How long have you been here?"

"Oh, where do we live. Mörfelder Landstrasse."

"Which city are we in?"

"Cassel—here Cassel—no, Frankfurt . . ."

"What kind of a building are you in?"

"That is . . . oh God. . . . Fifty-one . . . so fifty-one."

"What brought you here?"

"I actually don't know that—so fifty-one, 1851 . . ."

"What do you mean by that?"

"June fifty-one and . . ."

"Who are the people in your neighborhood?"

"Also in Mörfelder Landstrasse or . . .?"

"Who are the people in your neighborhood?"

"Oh, I don't even know the people at all . . ."

"Where were you eight days ago?"

"Eight days ago? They say I can't remember."

"Where were you a month ago?"

"Yes, that I can't say."

"Where were you last Christmas?"

"Christmas."

"Where were you last Christmas?"

"Yes, I can't tell you that so precisely. . . . Fifty-one. . . . I still have to remember that first."

"Are you sad?"

"Oh always, mostly not; it happens that one sometimes has courage."

"Are you sick?"

"Oh, I can't actually say. I'm sorry enough when I . . . as I said . . . oh God . . ."

"Are you persecuted?"

"Oh no, by God no."

"Are you mocked?"

"Oh no, I definitely could not say that."

"Do you hear voices?"

"Yes, you've already said that to me."

"Do you hear voices?"

"Oh yes, so, humming perhaps."[2]

"What hums?"

"Oh, it doesn't occur to me like that."

"Do you see shapes?"

"No, not at all."

"Who am I?"

"Oh, I already know."

"Who am I?"

In a whining tone Auguste D. answers, "I can't really say."

"Who am I?"

"Oh . . . oh . . ."

"Address me. What did you call me earlier? If you could just give me a bit of a hint."

"Doc . . . doctor."

"What am I?"

"Doctor."

Alzheimer was called to a patient who suddenly became agitated. An hour later he returned to Auguste D. Again he showed her various objects, which she named without touching them:

*Notebook*: "Book."

*Two-mark piece*: "Two marks."

*Pencil*: "Pencil."

*Purse*: "Purse."

*Sleeve*: "Sleeve."

*Knife*: "Knife."

*Handkerchief*: "Handkerchief."

*Newspaper page*: "Newspaper."

*Boot*: "Boot."

*Key*: "Key."

*Notebook*: "Notebook."

*Bunch of keys*: "Keys."

*Steel nib pen*: "Steel nib pen."

Dr. Alzheimer pointed to the steel nib pen: "What does one do with this?"

"One can write with it."

*Pocketwatch*: "Clock."

"What time is it now?" He indicated the clock face.

"Eight minutes before 2 o'clock, I mean, it would have been earlier: quarter to four, quarter to five, ah of course!"

Alzheimer indicated the Roman numeral II on the clock face: "What is the name of the number that my little finger is pointing to now?"

"Twenty!" Auguste D. pointed to the nurse and asks, "Who is that? A young lady?"

A patient with her hair down, animatedly gesticulating and noisy, was carried through the main room. Dr. Alzheimer asked Auguste D., "What is wrong with this person?"

"That is the hair . . ."

"What is wrong with this person?"

"Cheerful . . ."

Dr. Alzheimer did not want to overtax Auguste D., so he paused. Suddenly Auguste D. said, directly and in a clear voice, "But I don't want to know anything about thefts, I've heard nothing about them."

Dr. Alzheimer continued his examination, although things had become unsettled in the main room.

"Are you married?"

"I believe that I am married."

"Are you married?"

"Certainly, I have a fifty-two-year-old daughter in Berlin."

"How old are you?"

"Fifty-six."

"And your daughter is supposed to be fifty-two years old?"

"Fifty-three, no fifty-four."

"If you are fifty-six years old then your daughter cannot, of course, be fifty-two years old."

"Fifty-three, right, is what she . . ."

Alzheimer repeats the question again.

"I'm so nervous, fifty-three is what I am."

Dr. Alzheimer checked her skills in arithmetic. She solved simple arithmetic problems correctly:

"7 + 7?"

"14."

"10 − 8?"

"2."

"5 × 5?"

"55, oh no . . ."

"23 × 3?"

"I can't do that so quickly, at the moment I can't read that!"

"2 × 2?"

"4 . . . that, of course, is certain?"

"33 × 3?"

"9."

"6 × 6?"

"36."

"5 × 5?"

No answer.

"6 × 6?"

"36."

"8 × 8?"

"64."

"7 × 7?"

"I'm just nervous, I can't help myself."

"10 × 10?"

"100."

"20 − 10?"

"10."

"30 + 20?"

"50."

"5 × 5?"

"25."

"7 × 7?"

"44."

"8 − 5?"

"3."

"3 × 3?"

"7 × 3 I said . . ."

Then he checked the alphabet and the names of the months. "Recite the alphabet." Auguste D. fluently named the letters *A* through *J* and then went silent.

"Keep going."

"Oh please, I'm not dressed for it." She fiddled around with her nightshirt.

"Recite the alphabet."

Again she fluently listed the letters from *A* to *J*.

"Go on."

Auguste D. said nothing.

"Don't other letters come after *J*?"

"I don't know any more."

"Do you know the names of the months?"

Auguste D. said nothing.

"January—how does it go after that?"

"I cannot remember anything."

A physical examination was impossible that day because Auguste D. struggled violently against it, so Alzheimer turned again to other tasks in the clinic. In the afternoon Auguste D. lay in the big main room; in the evening she became unruly. She ran around the room wailing and grabbed other patients' faces so that they, too, became agitated. Dr. Nitsche, the doctor on duty, appeared.

"Oh, excuse me, doctor," she said, adding, as she so often did when she was excited, "and please don't take offense."

She did not answer the question of what one should not take offense at. Auguste D. was put in isolation, where she busied herself with the bedding. She told the doctor who looked after her, "Oh, doctor, don't take offense."

She was nervous and sat in bed with a helpless expression. Soon afterward she pushed doggedly toward the door: "Oh, I just want to get out." She pointed to the wall: "Who is here?"

"That is a wall," answered Dr. Nitsche and pointed to the bed. "What is this?"

"That is a bed."

After two hours she became calmer and was placed back in the main room. The same evening, Dr. Alzheimer continued his examination, handing Auguste D. a pencil and paper. At the top of the page he recorded the date. He later marked her answers with the numbers 1 through 7.

"What is your name?"

"May."

"Write your name down."

She wrote, "May."

"Write something."

She wrote something illegible.

"Who are you?"

"Mrs. D."

"Write it down."

She wrote, "Mrs. D." and read aloud, "Auguste D."

Alzheimer pointed to the word "Mrs."

"What is that word?"

"Yes, Mrs. Auguste D."

"Where is 'Auguste' written?"

Auguste D. did not react. Dr. Alzheimer wrote the word "garden" on the left margin of the page.

Auguste D. wrote, "Mrs. D."

Alzheimer repeated the request to write something.

Again, Auguste D. wrote something illegible.

"Write a 5."

She wrote, "Mrs."

"Write an 8."

She wrote, "Augufe."

Dr. Alzheimer turned the pencil upside down in her hand. At first she made several attempts to write with the upside-down pencil, then used it properly.

Alzheimer could not get the case of Auguste D. out of his mind. He remembered cases of age-induced feeble-mindedness that he had observed years before in much older patients. At that time he assumed that senile dementia could be triggered by the thickening of the blood vessels of the brain, or atherosclerosis.

In 1898 Alzheimer published an article about it, "Dementia Senilis and Brain Diseases Based on Atheromatous Vessel Disease," in the *Monatsschrift für Psychiatrie* (*Monthly Journal of Psychiatry*). He believed that atheromatous degeneration was responsible for the emergence of senile brain atrophy, which he therefore called arteriosclerotic brain atrophy. However, he wondered whether such changes could occur earlier in life, between ages fifty and sixty.

Several years before, Alzheimer had examined a case similar to that of Auguste D. During the autopsy and subsequent examination of the brain he had found signs of shrinkage of certain brain cells, called ganglial cells, but only minor arteriosclerotic changes in the vessels.

At that time he suspected a genetic predisposition, as well as a weakness of the central nervous system, that might result in early deterioration of the ganglial cells. However, this single case provided insufficient evidence; further examinations were needed to confirm his suspicions.

Auguste D. was the patient Alzheimer had been waiting for. He turned again to the notes that Dr. Nitsche made on November 26, 1901, the day Auguste D. was admitted.

As her date of birth Nitsche had entered "May 16, 1850," maiden name "H." Both her next of kin and Auguste D. herself had named Cassel as her birthplace. As it happened, Alzheimer's grandfather, Johann Alzheimer, also was from Cassel and had been a teacher there. When Auguste D.

started school, his grandfather was fifty-nine years old; it was therefore very likely that she had been Johann Alzheimer's student.

Alzheimer reviewed the admission sheet.

Admission number 7139
   *Name*: D., née H.
   *Given Name*: Auguste
   *Place of Birth*: Cassel
   *Home*: Prussia
   *Last Residence*: Frankfurt am Main, Mörfelder Landstrasse
   *Year and Day of Birth*: May 16, 1850
   *Marital Status*: Married
   *Religious Confession*: Reformed
   *Status or Profession*: Railway clerk's wife

The duration of illness Dr. Alzheimer entered himself: "half a year." To the question, "Are father and mother related to each other?" he answered, "No." There were nervous illnesses on her mother's side, and Auguste D. was not born out of wedlock. Next to the heading "Other Causes of Illness" he put "arteriosclerosis." The form of illness he labeled "arteriosclerotic brain atrophy" but marked the entry with a question mark. It also emerged from the admission sheet that Auguste D. had never been in legal trouble and had never been in a mental institution.

For the question, "Will the patient be cared for at own expense, first class, second class, third class, or at public expense third class?" Dr. Alzheimer underlined with his feather pen, "expense, third class." As form of illness, he wrote, "simple mental disorder."

On November 26, 1901, Nitsche had elicited a very thorough case history. According to his notes, Auguste D.'s mother had suffered from convulsions since menopause; however, during the attacks she did not drop objects that she held in her hands, nor did she lose consciousness. She had died of pneumonia at age sixty-four. The father had been healthy but died young, ostensibly from a "carbuncle on the neck." Auguste D.'s three siblings were in good health; no alcoholism or mental disorders were apparent in the family.

Auguste D.'s husband reported that his wife had always been healthy and had never had a serious illness. He said that they had been happily and harmoniously married since 1873. Auguste had had one daughter and had had no miscarriages. Her husband described his wife as constantly hard working and orderly; at most she was somewhat excitable and nervous but otherwise "rather amicable." She drank no alcohol, and there was no sexually transmitted disease in the family.

According to the husband's statement, Auguste D. had been quite normal until March 1901. On March 18, 1901, she suddenly claimed that he had gone for a walk with a female neighbor. This completely groundless assertion was the first thing that struck him. From that moment on Auguste had been full of mistrust about him and this neighbor. Shortly thereafter the husband noted a decline in her memory. Two months later, in May, she made obvious mistakes in food preparation for the first time and became restless, wandering aimlessly through the apartment. She increasingly neglected her housework; her condition deteriorated more and more. She then claimed "constantly" that a carter, who often came into the house, wanted somehow to harm her.

Conversations she overheard she took to be about herself. No language or speech disorders, or even signs of paresis, had emerged. Recently she had spoken frequently of death and had become agitated, especially in the mornings, when she trembled, rang the neighbors' doorbells, and slammed doors shut. She was never violent. Shortly before being admitted to the hospital she had hidden all sorts of objects, throwing the house into disorder.

For Alzheimer it was easy to understand that under these circumstances her husband could no longer cope and, on November 25, 1901, he had brought his wife to the institution. The family doctor had noted in large script on the admittance note,

> Mrs. Auguste D., wife of the railway clerk Mr. Carl D., Mörfelder Landstrasse, has been suffering for a long time from weakness of memory, persecution mania, sleeplessness, restlessness. She is unable to perform any physical or mental work. Her condition (chronic brain paresis) needs treatment from the local mental institution.

During the examination Alzheimer built a close and trusting relationship with Auguste D. His interest in her developed in part because of their shared hometown, Cassel. But Alzheimer also recognized very quickly that the case could prove to be of great scientific importance. He therefore arranged for a precise documentation of the course of the illness. He instructed the clinic photographer to take a number of pictures of Auguste D., including portrait photos.

Many photographs from June 1902 have been preserved. In one Auguste D. sits on a bench; in another she is in bed. On October 20, 1902, she was again photographed in bed.

In November 1902 a particularly impressive portrait emerged, a photo that almost a hundred years later, in 1997, was sent around the world. Auguste D. sits in her bed, turned to the side, with bent legs. She has full, long, dark brown hair; it hangs down both sides of her face in plaited strands. Her face is heavily wrinkled in the forehead and under the eyes; the folds alongside her nose are very prominent. Her face is thin, the exposed left ear rather large.

Auguste D. looks out blankly; she appears calm. Her well-groomed hands, with their strikingly long fingers, are folded over her knees. Auguste D. wears institutional clothing, a white nightshirt buttoned at the front.

Alzheimer developed the treatment plan himself. He prescribed baths for Auguste D. Alzheimer had done extensive work on the therapeutic value of warm and mild baths that extend over several hours, even days, and soothe agitated patients. A famous colleague, Emil Kraepelin, director of the Psychiatric Clinic in Heidelberg (and later Alzheimer's boss for a time), was also a champion of balneotherapy and climatology, which he had described in his 1896 textbook for students and doctors.

The initial treatment for insomnia was dietary. For patients with chronic illnesses and those with strong constitutions, extensive outdoor activity, exercise, and massage were prescribed, but strenuous physical exertions can cause sleeplessness in those who are easily excited or have recently become ill. For such patients, extended lukewarm baths with simultaneous cooling of the head and moist wrappings were preferred. Treating the head with weak electrical currents (galvanization) seemed appropriate to the physicians in some cases, as did hypnotic suggestion.

Often patients showed great improvement with the introduction of afternoon rest, light, early dinners, the avoidance of reading in the evening, abstention from tea and coffee, evening bowel evacuations, regular bedtimes, and extensive airing of the bedroom.

Alcohol was administered in mild doses. The doctors used sedatives only in emergencies—in cases of great fear or acute pain, for example—because it is difficult to reaccustom patients to natural sleep. In cases of extreme agitation refractory to other means, when rapid calming is necessary, chloroform was used.

In the treatment of Auguste D. and many other troubled patients, sedatives were very useful. Such patients were given 2 to 3 grams of chloral hydrate, a sedative that induced a longer-lasting, restful sleep. If the patient could not tolerate chloral hydrate, paraldehyde, an unpleasant-smelling and -tasting colorless liquid developed in 1883, could be administered. In small doses of 5 grams—which one can safely increase two- or threefold—it effects a long, deep, restful sleep, akin to natural sleep.

Amylene hydrate had certain advantages over paraldehyde; later sulphonal, tetronal, and somnol were used. The legendary Veronal (barbital), a barbituric acid preparation developed by Merck and Bayer, was still being tested on animals at this time and was not made available for patients for several years.

In February 1902 Auguste D. suffered from constant restlessness and anxious confusion. She approached each day with such a negative attitude that examining her became impossible. Consequently, she spent the entire day, and often the evening, in the bath. At night she was usually put in an isolation room because she could not fall asleep in the main ward; she went to other patients' beds and woke them. In a private room, after a longer or shorter period of persistent wandering about, she fell asleep.

Alzheimer noted that she would never lie properly in her bed and did not use the bedding correctly. She covered herself with pillows and huddled on the feather quilt.

When she was calm during the day, she was placed in the open ward. During rounds, she approached the doctor with a helpless expression and used only empty phrases: "Oh, good day—so?" or "What would you like then?"

For a while she believed she was at home and receiving guests. Then she said, "My husband will be here shortly!" But she could not continue the scene and turned away, ran about aimlessly, and fiddled with her bedding. When the staff attempted to restrain her, she began to cry, moan, and voice her indignation, using meaningless words and expressions.

Alzheimer saw Auguste D. almost daily during his rounds and during the weekly rounds with the clinic director, Dr. Sioli. Her diet was good, but the long conversations he could conduct with her three months earlier were no longer possible.

Alzheimer's last entry in the files of Auguste D. dates from June 1902:

Auguste D. continues to be hostile, screams, and lashes out when one wants to examine her. She also screams spontaneously, often for hours, so that she has to be kept in bed. As far as food is concerned, she no longer keeps to the regular mealtimes. A boil has formed on her back.

Alzheimer's last conversation with Auguste D. is well documented:
"Good day, Mrs. D."
"Oh, begone; I—cannot say—that."
Her agitation manifested itself in aimless wandering, purposeless activity, and especially loud wailing and screaming, which for several weeks appeared paroxysmal and lasted for several hours. Auguste D. appeared in a state of tremendous fear and called out, "Oh God—oh God—Heinrich!"

## 2. *Alois Alzheimer's Ancestry, Childhood, and Youth*

The ancestors of Alois Alzheimer, some of whom also spell their name "Alsheimer," came from the Franconian region of the Spessart.

In the mid-eighteenth century few strangers strayed into the densely wooded, low mountain range; the locals based their livelihood on the forest, whose wood they turned into staves. The importance of mining, particularly of copper and silver, eventually dwindled, and the numerous glassworks folded. Nevertheless, these hard-working and religious people stayed in their homeland, to which they had close ties, and were content.[1]

One of the first members of the Alzheimer family about whom there is a registry office certificate is Alois Alzheimer's great-grandfather, Michael Alzheimer, born in 1757 in Rengersbrunn. Rengersbrunn is a few kilometers north of Lohr am Main and today has about 160 inhabitants. It still has its agricultural character; the main source of income is the forest.

Old documents tell us, "The occupants of Rengersbrunn had it hard, and their work was hard." Already in the Middle Ages Rengersbrunn had become a place of pilgrimage to the Virgin Mary, and a charming legend has grown up around it:

It was in the time around 1460; Rengersbrunn consisted of a few houses. A shepherd tended his flock near the King's Well. The shepherd's dog crawled into a nearby hazelnut bush, and the sheep assembled all around it; the shepherd wanted to drive the herd farther on, but the herd and the dog could not be moved. After he had searched through the bush he found a life-size image, carved out of wood, of the mother of God with the Christ child on her arm. The discovery aroused understandable interest. The image was brought to what was at that time the only church in the vicinity, in Burgsinn. Because it was too tall for the chosen place, the bottom of the statue was cut off. It was then that the wonder occurred: On the next day the image stood, intact again, at the

King's Well. The statue was taken back to the Burgsinn parish church, and the mysterious disappearance and the discovery at the old place were repeated.[2]

The deeply pious Spessart peasants saw a sign from heaven in this story and built a small chapel at the King's Well. At first only Catholics from the region made the pilgrimage to the small chapel, but soon they came from near and far. Numerous donations supported the building of the pilgrimage church.

Like most of the other villagers, the Alzheimer family was deeply rooted in Franconia and held firmly to its Catholic beliefs. Believers come to the village today, as they have for centuries, with their many notes for the image of the holy Madonna, to find shelter and help.

On February 7, 1792, Michael Alzheimer married Margarethe Günther, also from Rengersbrunn, in Rengersbrunn's pilgrimage church. Five years later, in 1797, Johann Alzheimer, Alois Alzheimer's grandfather, was born; he lived in Rengersbrunn until 1825 in house number 6. In those days there were only twenty-two houses with twenty-two families.

Johann Alzheimer became a teacher and moved, in accordance with a government decree, to Cassel, a village in the Gelnhausen district in northwest lower Franconia.[3] Today Cassel, now Kassel, belongs to the municipality of Biebergemünd; what is now the city hall was in 1825 the newly built Cassel schoolhouse. The village chronicle reports, "After completion in fall 1825 the school was taken over by a teacher Alzheimer from Rengersbrunn, and in the same year Kassel got a second teacher."[4]

The chronicle also reveals that bureaucratic duties and functions were bound up with the primary teaching position. As a result, Johann Alzheimer also prepared deeds and other documents, for which he received the corresponding fees. He thus ended up with an annual salary of 810 marks, along with 90 marks for heating and a free apartment—a good income in those days. In 1825 Cassel's population numbered 905, of whom only 168 were men, largely because of the Napoleonic wars.

Two years after the move from Rengersbrunn to Cassel, Johann Alzheimer's wife, Crescentia, née Bachmann, had her first son, Karl Georg, on October 6, 1827. The second, Eduard, came into the world on March 22, 1830.

At first Johann taught both sons himself; then he sent them to the high school in Aschaffenburg. Karl Georg was a good student and while still at high school received a scholarship of 70 florins from the general school and study fund. After completing school he studied theology in Würzburg and later, as a Catholic priest, held the office of the First Prefect at the boys' seminary in Aschaffenburg. Karl Georg always remained close to his younger brother, Eduard.

Eduard was just as talented as his brother. In 1853, as a student of jurisprudence, he received a scholarship from the Friedrich Fund. He became a notary, and in Würzburg he married Eva Maria Sabina Busch in 1861.

In the next year Eduard moved to the Lower Franconian city of Marktbreit as First Royal Notary in the Royal District Court. He drew attention to himself in the local newspaper: "The undersigned begins his official activity on July 2 this year. . . . Marktbreit, June 24, 1862, Eduard Alzheimer, Royal Notary."[5]

Protestant minister R. Plochmann reported on the small Lower Franconian locale in his village chronicle of 1864:

Marktbreit was always and is still an important trade location with direct connections to the most highly regarded firms in the big trade and seaside towns of Germany, England, Holland, France and Belgium, Italy and America. . . . Trade is conducted mainly in colonial produce; precious woods; all kinds of metals; local and foreign, namely French, Hungarian, and Spanish wines; weaving materials and wools; and regional wholesale goods of all kinds.[6]

Eduard Alzheimer established his offices in a building that is still one of the most magnificent houses in town. The portal is crowned with a broken gable. Over the insignia of the Günter family the allegory of hope is prominently displayed. It is this to which the Latin inscription on the ledge refers: "*en Mea spes aeDes Certae aC paX arXq Ve beata*" ("See here my securely constructed dwelling place, my hope, place of peace, and happy bastion"). The capitalized letters of the Latin inscription, *MDCCXXV*, indicate the year of construction.

FIGURE 2.1 *The house in Marktbreit where Alois Alzheimer was born*

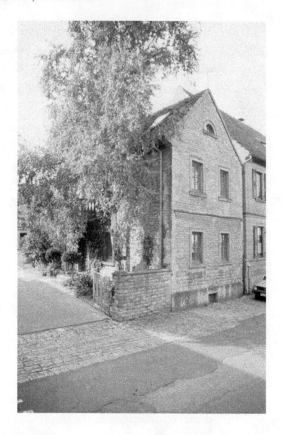

In these chambers Eduard Alzheimer certified a wide range of documents. A certificate from May 27, 1862, documents the beginning of the age of the railway:

> In cases of illness the town of Marktbreit will accommodate railway construction workers building the Marktbreit Section of the Royal Railroad to the Marktbreit town hospital. The town commits itself to admitting the railway workers to a maximum number of twenty-five patients, to care for them and have them medically treated. Daily rate per patient for care, medical treatment, and medicines: 39 Kreuter. A special compensation is paid for the consultation of a second or third doctor.[7]

Eduard Alzheimer and his family moved into an apartment not far

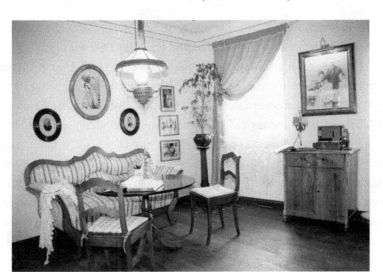

FIGURE 2.2    *The room where Alzheimer was born, now part of the museum*

from the offices, on the first floor of a large residential building at 336 Würzburgerstrasse. The house still stands today.

Great joy was followed by great suffering in July 1862 when Eduard's first son, Karl Eduard Sebastian, was born and his young mother died three weeks later at age twenty-six. On July 31, 1862, Eduard Alzheimer notified the town magistrate of the death of his wife, Eva Maria Sabina: "Time of entry of death: July 26, 1862, 7 o'clock in the evening; cause of death: puerperal fever, aged twenty-six years and two months. She leaves behind a child, three weeks old."

After a year of mourning Eduard married the sister of his deceased wife a practice that was not unusual at the time. The registry office notes, "On October 1, 1863, Theresia Busch, the sister of the deceased Eva Maria Sabina, and Eduard Alzheimer, Royal Notary, entered into the bond of marriage."

Theresia did not want to live in the house in which her sister had died because the thought of giving birth there made her uneasy, so the Alzheimers moved at the beginning of 1864 into 273 Würzburgerstrasse, a smaller house with a graceful exterior.

What is special about this house is a tubular notch in the brickwork that was knocked into the wall during construction to allow an existing birch tree to grow unhindered. A birch still graces this house today. It is the house in which Alois Alzheimer was born on June 14, 1864, the second son of Royal Notary Eduard Alzheimer and his wife, Theresia.

On December 19, 1995, the eightieth anniversary of Alois Alzheimer's death, the house was donated to the public as a memorial after being acquired by American pharmaceutical company Eli Lilly, restored under the direction of Ulrike Maurer, and furnished as a museum and conference center.

The mother of the newborn Alois survived the birth without complications. Fortunately, the puerperal fever that killed Eva Maria Sabina claims fewer victims today. In 1847 Hungarian obstetrician Ignaz Semmelweis demonstrated the connection between dirt and the transmission of illness. He worked in a Vienna hospital where the annual mortality rate for women was 10 percent, in some months as high as 20 percent, whereas in a neighboring maternity home run by nuns the rate was less than 3 percent. The women died predominantly of septicemia.

It struck Semmelweis that the maternity home was cleaner than the hospital because under the rules of their order, the nuns were obliged to maintain personal cleanliness. The doctors in the hospital, on the other hand, operated in dirty suits and did not think it necessary to keep their clothing clean; it would only get filthied with blood and pus anyway. Furthermore, the doctors often came to the sick ward directly from the dissection room. Semmelweis instructed his co-workers to wash their hands before every examination with soap and a chlorine–lime solution. He thus reduced the mortality rate at the hospital to 1.2 percent.

In the "Private Announcements" section of the *Marktbreiter Wochenblatt* (*Marktbreit Weekly*) of Wednesday, June 15, 1864, the happy father announced, "Tuesday, June 14, 1864, our son Aloysius was born. I inform my dear relatives and friends and acquaintances."

The announcement of the joyful event did not fit the appearance of the newspaper at that time. For the past several months the paper had been printed with a black border of mourning because of the sudden death of his majesty, King Maximilian II of Bavaria, whose successor was the legendary King Ludwig II.

In this small, predominantly Protestant Franconian town Alois Alzheimer was baptized as a Catholic in his parents' home on July 3, 1864. In the baptismal register, available in the Würzburg Episcopal archive, one can still read,

Aloysius—second child of second marriage—*midwife*: the same—*Father*: Eduard Alzheimer, Royal Notary—*Residence*: house number 273—*Father's Name and Profession*: Alzheimer Notary—*Date of Birth*: 14.6.1864, around 4 in the morning—*Baptism*: 3 July 1864 in parental home—*Officiating Priest*: Canon Mr. Ignatz Ruhland in Würzburg and *godfather*: Chaplain Mr. Aloys Alzheimer of Sulzfeld.[8]

After the birth of little Alois, Eduard Alzheimer and his wife prepared themselves for a long stay in Marktbreit. In the same year Alzheimer bought a piece of meadow land—only with proof of land ownership could he become a burgher of the municipality—and acquired, for a fee of 25 florins, the rights of a burgher of the town of Marktbreit. That he was also accepted into the small-town society is demonstrated by his election in 1870 to treasurer of the music and singing club; he became president of the club in 1872. In the same year this highly regarded burgher was authorized as plenipotentiary of the municipality.

Consequently, Alois grew up without a care in the world. There is a photograph from his childhood, probably from 1866, that shows him on his mother's lap. As an adult, Dr. Alzheimer told his children the following anecdote:

I remember clearly a maid in Marktbreit whom we children loved very much. She first became fascinating for me, however, when a thunderstorm was approaching. Then she always disappeared into her room and took from her bedpost a small linen sack in which she had collected bread crusts. In no time she crawled under the bed and chewed noisily on the old crusts until the storm passed. I lay down on the floor in front of the bed to observe her closely, and despite my curiosity I was overcome by the creeps.[9]

From 1870 to 1874 the gifted boy attended the Catholic school in Marktbreit, yet his father did not see further schooling in Marktbreit as satisfactory. The fact that Marktbreit and the surroundings had seen a kind of diaspora for Catholic families also suggested that the family should leave Marktbreit. Eduard often discussed this question with his older brother,

FIGURE 2.3 *Alzheimer (at right) at age 2 with his mother, Theresia, and two of his siblings, Karl and Johanna*

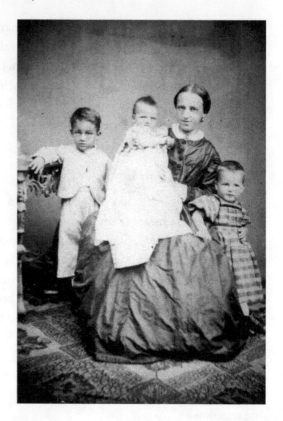

Georg, who at this time was a priest in Grosswallstadt and had applied for a parish in Aschaffenberg.

The ten-year-old Alois was the first in the family to move to Aschaffenburg: His father and uncle got lodgings for him in a guest house so that from 1874 on he could attend the Royal Humanistic Gymnasium.

Meanwhile, five more children were born at 273 Würzburgerstrasse through 1875: two daughters and three sons. Karl and Alois were followed by Anna Johanna Barbara Sabina, born December 19, 1865, who later became a nun. Eduard Roman, born on February 17, 1867, later became a pharmacist; after him, on New Year's Day of 1870, came Max Theodor Alexander, who later became a priest. His younger sister, Maria Crescentia Elisabeth, was born on June 26, 1872. The last child of the Royal Notary and his second wife, Theresia, was Johann Alfred, who was born on September 20, 1875, and later became director of an agricultural school.

The decision to leave Marktbreit was finalized by 1878, and the family made the necessary preparations. On July 10, 1878, Royal Notary Eduard Alzheimer authenticated his last document in Marktbreit.

In mid-1878 the Alzheimers and their seven children moved to Aschaffenburg, initially living at Landingstrasse until Eduard Alzheimer purchased a magnificent house from the mid-eighteenth century in Dalbergstrasse, opposite the town hall.

Alois and his brothers attended the renowned Royal Humanistic Gymnasium, the same school that their father and their uncle Georg had already attended. Alois passed the final exam on July 14, 1883, with the following evaluation:

Among his written examinations it is chiefly the German essay, through the sensible handling of which he had already distinguished himself during his student years, that shows maturity of judgment and skillfulness in presentation. In oral translations from both ancient languages he also shows largely correct understanding of what is read and knows how to discuss the relevant content satisfactorily. His achievements in French were more modest, those in mathematics and history good. This student displayed outstanding knowledge of the natural sciences, with which he occupied himself with a particular liking throughout his entire high school career.

During his residence in the school he behaved with decency and evidenced a cast of mind turned positively to the good. Of course, just this was lacking insofar as he belonged as an office-bearer to a school association that bore the name "Abituria" and set itself the task of preparing a festive departure from the Gymnasium. His diligence was particularly praiseworthy in the subjects that especially interested him.

In particular, after the exams and tests given in the upper classes, his knowledge can be marked as follows:

*In religion*: very good,

*in German*: very good,

*in Latin*: good,

*in Greek*: satisfactory,

*in French*: satisfactory,

*in mathematics and physics*: good,
*in history*: good,
*in gymnastics*: excused.

In 1882, a year before Alois's final exam, he suffered a heavy blow: His mother died at age forty-two. His father remarried, to Martha Katharina Maria, née Geiger, who gave him a last child in 1884, his daughter Eugenia Alzheimer. Eduard Alzheimer was always a strict father but took great joy and pride in the thought that each of his children would amount to something.

## 3. Student of Medicine

With his high school diploma under his belt, in the summer of 1883 the nineteen-year-old Alois Alzheimer had to decide what to study. It had been a family tradition for the Alzheimers to devote themselves to serving humanity; many had become teachers and priests. As a notary, Alois's father had almost daily contact with the people in his neighborhood, just as his uncle Georg had had as a priest. On the other hand, there was Alois's predilection for the natural sciences. But choosing to study the natural sciences would have left him wanting for human contact.

None of his ancestors had entered the medical profession, but in it Alois saw a meaningful way to combine his inclinations. As the big brother of so many children, he probably also sensed the joy of being there for others and the desire to help, traits that were so evident throughout his life.

He also had to decide where to study. His older brother, Karl (actually his half-brother, although they resembled one other so closely that each could be mistaken for the other), wanted to bring him to Würzburg, where he had returned for the 1882–83 winter semester after earlier studies in Würzburg, Strassburg, and Munich. In Würzburg Karl Alzheimer led the Franconian Corps fraternity as first office-bearer. Also, Würzburg's proximity to Aschaffenburg meant that Alois could maintain close contact with his family; one could travel by rail from Aschaffenburg to Würzburg in a short time.

### Berlin: The Mecca of Medicine

His ambitious father wanted Alois to study in Berlin, however, and advised him to begin his medical studies there, not least because Berlin was at that time considered the Mecca of medicine.

In Berlin, Rudolf Virchow dominated the medical establishment. His international reputation as a pathologist was based on his work in cellular pathology and oncology. Virchow's ideas revolutionized nineteenth-century medicine. Not only was he the leader of his specialty, but he also mastered a variety of other fields. He believed it important to think in terms of practical outcomes and to place science in the service of such goals. For this reason, Berlin in the second half of the nineteenth century was considered a modern city, particularly in terms of public health.

Virchow exemplified the German scientist. The diversity of his interests is demonstrated by his interest in archaeology. In 1883, excavations in Mycenae stimulated the almost sixty-year-old Heinrich Schliemann to take up work in Troy again. It was with the assistance of Rudolf Virchow that Schliemann succeeded in finding historic Troy.

Virchow was just as strongly engaged in politics: As one of the founders of the German Progress Party, at the beginning of the 1870s Virchow coined the term *Kulturkampf* (cultural struggle) and for more than ten years, as a member of parliament, was a political opponent of Bismarck.

Along with Rudolf Virchow, Robert Koch helped Berlin attain its scientific reputation. Koch made the Royal Department of Health in Berlin one of the most highly regarded places for bacteriological research. In 1882—shortly before Alzheimer arrived in Berlin—Koch discovered *Mycobacterium tuberculosis*, the bacterium that causes tuberculosis. Largely eradicated from Western countries today, tuberculosis was at that time one of the greatest maladies threatening human life. Around 1880 one in seven deaths in Germany was attributable to tuberculosis, and between ages fifteen and forty this disease accounted for half of all deaths. Koch's discovery and the subsequent treatment led to a significant increase in human life expectancy.

In 1883 Koch set another medical milestone when, on a research expedition in India, he found *Vibrio cholerae*, the cholera pathogen, and demonstrated its spread through dirty drinking water. Koch was thus the first to offer proof of the microbial origin of a human infectious disease, and through this accomplishment he became world-famous overnight. He was awarded the Nobel prize in 1905.

The desire to be near these great doctors led Alois Alzheimer to make the leap from provincial Aschaffenburg to the empire's capital city. He began his medical studies in Berlin in the 1883–84 winter semester and was entered in the official registry of personnel and students of the Royal Friedrich Wilhelm University in Berlin for the winter semester from October 15, 1883, to March 15, 1884:

*Name of the Student*: Alois Alzheimer
*Place of Birth or Fatherland*: Bavaria
*Study*: Med.
*Police District*: NW
*House No.*: 7
*Street Name*: Neustädtische Kirch

He attended lectures and dissection exercises in anatomy by Prof. Heinrich Wilhelm Gottfried von Waldeyer. He took zoology from Prof. Karl Eduard Martens, inorganic experimental chemistry from Prof. Adolf Pinner, the botany of nonflowering plants from Prof. August Wilhelm Eichler, and selected lectures on plant physiology from Max Westermaier.

Waldeyer's anatomy lectures appealed to him above all. At that time, this pathologist had published an article, "The Development of Carcinoma," in Rudolf Virchow's journal *Archiv für die Pathologische Anatomie und Physiologie und für die Klinische Medizin* (*Archive of Pathological Anatomy and Physiology and Clinical Medicine*).

Waldeyer argued that cancer cells developed from normal cells that grew excessively and increased through cell division. In Waldeyer's opinion, the emergence of the primary tumor occurred exclusively as insistent growth into the surrounding tissue. The spread of secondary tumors, or metastasis, occurred through the circulatory or lymphatic pathways or other bodily fluids. Waldeyer's theory of the emergence and spread of cancer grounded modern cancer research and the operative methods of treatment derived from it and corresponds to today's knowledge.

Carl Westphal taught psychiatry at the famous Charité. Together with his predecessor Wilhelm Griesinger, he introduced cerebral pathology into psychiatry and was appointed to the chair of psychiatry in Berlin in 1865. Westphal taught about compulsive phenomena and agoraphobia (fear of open spaces), but he was primarily a specialist in pathological anatomy and tried to investigate brain damage in psychoses. It was in the psychiatry lectures that Alois Alzheimer encountered for the first time—and was immediately fascinated by—the nonrestraint principle developed by John Conolly of Great Britain, a "free treatment of the insane without the hitherto usual drastic measures of restraint."[1]

The Catholic-educated student from the country had little taste for the various stimuli that city of Berlin had to offer; he felt the tug of his

Franconian homeland. After the winter semester he returned his books to the Royal University Library on March 7, 1884, and on March 1, 1884, for a fee of 12 marks and 50 pfennigs, he received his leaving certificate:

> We, rector and senate of the Royal Friedrich Wilhelm University of Berlin, state with this leaving certificate that Mr. Alois Alzheimer, born at Marktbreit, son of the notary Alzheimer, prepared for academic study at the *Gymnasium* at Aschaffenburg, was, on the basis of this diploma, enrolled at our institution on October 16, 1883, was resident here as a student until the end of the winter semester 1883–84, and studied medicine. During this residence the above-named regularly attended the lectures attested to in the presented reports.[2]

## Corps Student in Würzburg

In the summer of 1884 Alois Alzheimer began his second semester in Würzburg. He knew the diocesan town from his childhood; his father had studied there and married the mother of Alois's older brother, Karl. Because of his family's ties to Würzburg, he enrolled in the medical school there on April 23, 1884, and initially resided at Badgasse 1.

His older brother, Karl, had little difficulty recruiting Alois for his fraternity, the Franconian Corps. The summer semester of 1884 was a hard one for the fraternity. After the university's 300th anniversary in the 1882 summer semester, the number of active corps brothers members had dropped from thirty to four, so new students were needed to keep the corps alive.

Alois Alzheimer was happy to be accepted and eagerly joined in. He contributed the experience he had gained through activities with the high school association Abituria, for which he had received censure in his diploma. Alois enjoyed the fraternity life in his second semester, went to few lectures, changed his residence several times, and, at the end of the summer semester on July 25, 1884, was accepted into the select corps of the Franconia. He was an enthusiastic and engaged Franconian, and many different ranks were later conferred on him; the family tradition Karl founded in the Franconians was continued, after Alois, by Eduard, who was accepted into the select corps on June 11, 1890.[3]

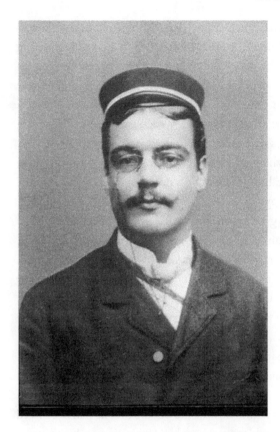

FIGURE 3.1 *Alois Alzheimer in 1884 as a member of the Würzburg Franconian Corps*

As a student in Würzburg, Alois Alzheimer launched into far more social than academic activities, including fencing. During one fencing bout he sustained a huge gash on his face. The scar extended from the left side of the lower eyelid over the entire left cheek, bordering the mustache in the form of a bow. This is probably why, with few exceptions, Alzheimer let himself be photographed only from the right side.

During the 1884 summer semester he attended only a chemistry course; these lectures on the chemistry of metals with Prof. Johann Wislicenus cost 30 marks.

In the winter semester of 1884–85 Alzheimer moved into a room at Inneren Graben 45 and began to devote himself more to his academic studies.[4] He attended the main lecture by Prof. Adolf Fick, a famous physiologist, after whom Fick's laws are named. Fick's laws allow for a macroscopic physical and mathematical description of diffusion.

More important for Alzheimer, however, was the contact with histology Prof. Alfred von Kölliker, who introduced him to the fascinating world of the microscope. In von Kölliker's institute worked famous researchers such as Alfonso Corti, who later won the Nobel prize, and Franz von Leydig. Both of them gave their names to organs and cell systems: Corti's organ, the sense organ in the auditory cochlea; and Leydig's cells, interstitial cells in the testes that secrete testosterone.

The close contacts Alzheimer developed during the microscopy course with von Kölliker later led him to devote his doctoral thesis and a traineeship to the art of microscopy.

Alzheimer would not give up on the natural sciences that he loved so much, so he attended lectures on physics by Prof. Friedrich Kohlrausch, pioneer of the theory of electricity after whom Kohlrausch's law is named. For the preliminary examination in medicine, the *Physikum*, Alzheimer needed still more courses in the natural sciences—physiology, zoology, and botany—and these he took with Julius von Sachs. Thus prepared, he effortlessly passed the *Physikum* at the end of the 1885 summer semester.[5]

Afterward Alzheimer indulged in a high-spirited student prank: Immediately after the examination he boarded the train from Würzburg to Aschaffenburg. Just before Aschaffenburg he put on white tails in the train compartment. His bow tie and the bow of the poodle that he had borrowed from a fraternity brother were deep red in color. Having arrived at the train station, he got into a coach drawn by four black horses and rode to his father's office with the poodle on his lap. In front of the office the coachman blew his horn, and in every floor of the surrounding houses at least one window opened. The surprised inhabitants of Aschaffenburg shook their heads. The family initially was embarrassed, but they soon laughed about Alois's prank.[6]

For the 1885–86 winter semester Alois Alzheimer lived at Johannitersgasse 5, and it was then that he began his medical studies in earnest. The clinical lectures and practical training drew his full attention. He attended lectures on general pathology and the clinical course of poisonings, as well as lectures by privatdozent Georg Matterstock on percussion and auscultation, which students at that time called the *Klopfkurs* ("percussion course").

Each of these lectures cost 20 to 30 marks per semester, quickly adding up to several hundred marks per semester. The lectures on forensic psychiatry especially fascinated Alzheimer. They were given by Prof. Hubert

Grashey, who since 1884 had occupied the psychiatry chair in Würzburg. When on June 13, 1886, King Ludwig II, together with his psychiatrist, von Gudden, drowned under mysterious circumstances in the Starnberg Sea, Grashey became von Gudden's successor and in 1886 took up the full professorship in psychiatry at Munich.

## A Semester in Tübingen

On October 20, 1886, Alois Alzheimer left the university in Würzburg to spend the 1886–87 winter semester studying at the Eberhard Karl University in Tübingen.

His father, Eduard, had issued him a document that granted his son permission to study in Tübingen and assumed responsibility for his maintenance. For a fee of 10 marks and 90 pfennigs, Alzheimer enrolled at the university on November 12, 1886, and found quarters at the hotel Prince Karl at 6C Hafengasse.[7]

Alzheimer had reached his seventh semester, and it was high time for him to dedicate himself more intensively to his medical studies. Things were harder in Swabia than in Franconia, as indicated by the documents concerning Alzheimer's time as a student in Tübingen. He attended six lectures and recitations: specialized pathology and therapy, the medical clinic, a course of lectures on fractures and dislocations, the surgery clinic, the theory and practice of birthing, and the obstetrics and gynecology course. He must have worked incredibly hard, because in this semester he took eight courses in just a few months.

However, there was also an associated Franconian fraternity in Tübingen. Despite his determination and sense of duty, Alzheimer did not distance himself from student life and participated in a number of traditional Tübingen student pranks. At 6 feet tall, he was what the Franconians called a "Prügel-Mannsbild," or "big brute"; his Swabian classmates respectfully called him an "enormous fellow" and described him as having a boisterous and occasionally unruly nature.

Once, after losing a bet, he swam across the Main River in winter. One night in Tübingen he made so much noise outside a police station that he was punished with a 3-mark fine, which he had to pay to the university cashier.[8] Such student pranks and tests of courage, designed to disconcert

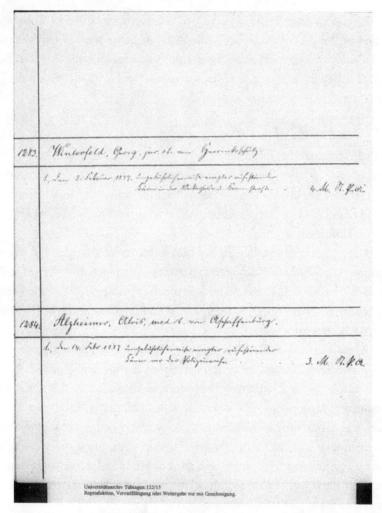

FIGURE 3.2  *Punishment records of Tübingen University from February 14,*
*1887. It reads, "Improper disturbance of the peace in front of the police station."*
*The penalty assessed is 3 marks.*

good citizens and institutions, were typical of student life of the time; punishment was more of an honor than a disgrace.

Perhaps Alzheimer saw things differently when he visited the Swabian
university town again twenty years later, in November 1906. Under the
auspices of the thirty-seventh assembly of the Southwest German Psychiatrists, he gave a talk called "A Peculiar Disease of the Cerebral Cortex"
on the Auguste D. case. As a result of this historic lecture, by the mid-

twentieth century one of the most malignant and widespread geriatric illness bore the name *Alzheimer's disease.*

## In Würzburg Again: The Doctoral Thesis

The influence of his brother Karl may have played a role in Alzheimer's decision to return to Würzburg for the summer semester of 1887 and finish his
studies there. But the more important reason probably was his predilection
for microscopy, the foundation of which had been laid by von Kölliker in
the winter semester of 1884–85.

The semesters in Würzburg were labor-intensive. Alzheimer attended eight lecture series in the summer semester, at a cost of 155 marks; at
this time he also started his doctoral thesis. The lectures covered the
fields of surgery, ophthalmology, gynecology, internal medicine, and
vaccination technique. In the summer semester he resumed his contact
with von Kölliker, with whom he studied embryology. Under Prof.
Philipp Stöhr he covered topographic anatomy. In 1887 von Kölliker or
Stöhr, or both, assigned Alois Alzheimer the topic of his doctoral thesis,
"On the Earwax Glands."[9]

Aristotle had already thought about the origin and composition of this
secretion of the human body. At that time, the common assumption was
that earwax was a waste product of brain activity. More recent studies had
ascribed it a protective function against various pests that could crawl into
the ear during sleep.

In Würzburg, ten years earlier, earwax plugs had brought the most important German psychiatrist of his time, Emil Kraepelin, an unprecedented
therapeutic triumph. He wrote about it in his memoirs: "I remember an old
woman whom I cured of a long-standing deafness through the removal of
hardened earwax plugging; she was so taken by this wonder that she performed a prayer of thanks on her knees."

In his thesis—a mere seventeen pages—which he completed in the
microscopy department of the Würzburg Anatomical Institute,
Alzheimer began by giving a historical overview of previous published
work on the topic. Physicians generally agreed on the anatomic structure
of the earwax glands, but there were contradictory opinions on the emergence of the glands and the outward openings of the glandular tubes.

Through his own investigations, the doctoral candidate came to the following conclusions:

1. The earwax glands emerge through the outgrowth of the external root sheath of the hair follicle.
2. In the newborn the sheaths still join in the hair follicles. But the ends slowly and gradually move higher on the hair follicle, emerging in adults on the open surface of the skin. For some the earlier relationship continues to obtain.

The last two pages of the thesis, on the emergence and significance of earwax and its composition, are particularly informative: "Earwax consists essentially of numerous fat granules and yellow-brown, irregular crumbs, as well as cells that potassium salt proves are fat-filled, undoubtedly originating in the sebaceous glands, and a chance addition of epidermal flakes and hair."

Typical of Alzheimer's scientific habits was his refusal to speculate; instead, he soberly remarks, "Whether some kind of special task really falls to earwax will not be considered here."

The accompanying histologic figures, which Alzheimer drew himself, are extraordinary, revealing a meticulous researcher skilled in producing pathohistologic drawings. In viewing the tables a specialist immediately sees that Alzheimer had found an area of medicine that allowed his gifts for observation, depiction, and description to flourish: the introduction of microscopy into psychiatry.

At the end of the thesis, for which Alzheimer received his medical doctorate in 1887, the medical candidate thanked his advisers:

It is for me a pleasant duty to thank Privy Councillor Prof. von Kölliker and Dr. Schulze for their friendly support. However, I am obliged to give special thanks to Dr. Stöhr, who at all times helped in the development of the topic that he entrusted to me with the greatest kindness and friendliness.

In winter semester of 1887–88 Alzheimer was no longer enrolled but nevertheless attended four lecture series on hygiene, outpatient clinics, eye clinics, and a surgical preparatory course. The book in which the courses he attended are entered shows no record of a psychiatry lecture.

In 1888 Alzheimer completed his examinations and made his final choice of profession. On May 12, 1888, he passed the state medical examination before the Würzburg medical examination commission with the grade "very good." On June 4, 1888, the Royal Bavarian State Ministry of the Interior for Church and School Affairs granted him a license to practice medicine for the territory of the German Empire.[10]

In Germany, 1888 was known as the Three-Kaiser Year, when grandson followed grandfather and father to the German throne. After the death of ninety-one-year-old Kaiser Wilhelm I on March 9, the ninety-nine-day reign of his seriously ill son, Friedrich III, began; Friedrich III died on June 15 of throat cancer, and his twenty-nine-year-old son, Wilhelm II, succeeded him as King of Prussia and German Kaiser.

On May 21, 1888, Friedrich III's throat cancer became a political issue that made medical history. The Imperial House had called in British throat specialist Morrell Mackenzie to treat the Crown Prince. Mackenzie took a small tissue sample of the throat tumor in question, which was handed over to Rudolf Virchow for histologic examination. Whereas the German surgeon recommended a "thorough eradication of the growth" "because of possible malignancies" and urged a speedy operation, the Briton held the illness to be noncancerous, even after hearing Virchow's opinion. When, despite sojourns at health spas and the efforts of numerous doctors, Friedrich died, the public criticism of Mackenzie, the "English swindler," escalated into nationalistic tirades of hate.

Of greater consequence for the history of medicine than this unpleasant argument was another event: In 1888 Sigmund Freud, who had studied at the Saltpêtrière in Paris with Jean Martin Charcot, translated a monograph by Hippolyte M. Bernheim into German.

In his monograph Bernheim defined the concept of suggestion according to a reflex model in which words alone introduce ideas to the brain, which believes them. When controlled reason is switched off by hypnosis, this "centripetal phenomenon" attempts to convert itself centrifugally—as sensation, image, or movement—into action. The suggestive therapy, or psychotherapy, consisted of using this automatism of the brain therapeutically. "The word alone is enough" was Bernheim's main methodological principle. He attempted to tackle all possible functional organ disorders with verbal suggestions and thereby brought curative ideas to his patients as a kind of hypnotist.

Thus a completely new field of psychiatry was opened up: clinical psychotherapy. In a few years Alois Alzheimer not only introduced the art of microscopy into psychiatry but also contributed to psychiatry's great interest in talking with patients, a contribution that found expression in his published accounts of such dialogues.

## 4. From Würzburg to Frankfurt

One well-known German psychiatrist of the time—they were called *Irrenärtze* (literally, loony-doctors, also called alienists) and referred to themselves as such—was Heinrich Hoffmann. He was born in Frankfurt in 1809. His mother died half a year after his birth, and four years later his father married the sister of his dead wife. Hoffmann studied medicine in Heidelberg and Halle and in Paris hospitals. The son of an architect, he became a doctor who treated the poor for free, an anatomist at the Senckenberg Institute in Frankfurt, and a pathologist; it was he who introduced the art of microscopy into histologic examinations.

For Europe the year 1848 was one of wide-ranging transformations, deep turbulence, great hopes, and equally great disappointments. Yet Hoffmann devoted all his energies to bringing about psychiatric reform; he left the political stage and in 1851 became the director of the Asylum for the Insane and Epileptic in Frankfurt. One of the predecessor clinics was a madhouse; after 1780 it was called *Kastenhospital* and was maintained by the city's charity organization. The "Asylum for the Epileptic" was added in 1815, and in 1833 the Asylum for the Insane and Epileptic emerged through an amalgamation under the control of a common Office for Social Services.

In 1859 Hoffmann wrote his first textbook and published it under the title *Beobachtungen und Erfahrungen über Seelenstörungen und Epilepsie in der Irrenanstalt zu Frankfurt am Main 1851 bis 1858* (*Observations and Experiences of Mental Disturbances and Epilepsy in the Institution for the Insane at Frankfurt am Main from 1851 to 1858*).[1]

Hoffmann's classification of the individual forms of psychiatric illness was remarkably clear and consistent with clinical experience of his day. His classifications included melancholia, mania, partial madness, general madness, imbecility (dementia), and epilepsy.

One of the most important psychiatric journals of the mid-nineteenth century, the *Allgemeine Zeitschrift für Psychiatrie und Psychisch-Gerichtliche*

*Medizin* (*General Journal of Psychiatry and Psychiatric-Forensic Medicine*), wrote of this work, "While reading this text one feels simultaneously spellbound and drawn in, as if walking through a beautiful park." Hoffmann's book is grippingly written and contains case histories that are readable and exciting, even for the layperson. He was a keen observer, one who well understood how to use his clinical experience both for himself and for the well-being of the patients entrusted to him.

Hoffmann very concretely divided the manias, characterized by a pathologically rapid flow of psychological processes, into acute manias, mania transitoria, mania simplex, mania religiosa, nymphomania and mania erotica, megalomania, and mania chronica. He remarked of megalomania that "this madness is nothing other than the confused and distorted mirror image of healthy psychological life." How little the book is geared toward instructions and explanations is conveyed by a conversation it reproduces between Hoffmann and a patient:

> The patient, in a period of calm delusion, greets Hoffmann courteously and says that now, fortunately, he will not go to Hell. When Hoffmann replies with a laugh, "Now that *is* fortunate!" the patient says, "Oh woe! Now you will have to go to hell after all." Then he adds with a serious, self-satisfied expression, "So today, then, the day of consecration is decided!"
> "Which day of consecration, Mr. N.?"
> "That on which I am consecrated as Christ!"
> "Is a consecration required for that?"
> "When you became a doctor, weren't you also consecrated?"
> "Sure, but according to scripture Christ was born the son of God; a consecration could not have made him that."

Hoffmann described the patient's reaction as follows: "Upon that the patient becomes indignant, stands up, and says he does not want to listen to my stupid prattle any longer."

In the nineteenth century two opposing schools of thought developed on the hotly disputed questions of the causes of mental illnesses, how they emerge, and how they were to be treated: the "psychicists" and the somaticists. The "psychicists" saw the causes and the possibilities for treatment in the mind; the somaticists saw them in the body.

Like many of his German colleagues, Hoffmann was no "psychicist." He did not want to "fill up sheets of paper by writing psychological paraphrases." He belonged unequivocally to the somaticists, who regarded mental illness as physically conditioned, and followed Wilhelm Griesinger, the professor of psychiatry in Berlin who, with his 1845 textbook *Pathology and Therapy of Psychic Illnesses*, had ushered in the natural scientific epoch of psychiatry.

The gist of Greisinger's theory resides in a well-known quote: "Mental illnesses are brain illnesses." He therefore attached great importance to neuropathology and made it the foundational science of a psychiatry oriented toward the natural sciences.

Hoffmann was also interested in autopsies and postmortem anatomic findings. As a somaticist he participated in many autopsies and himself carried out seventy-three of them in seven years: "Of these seventy-three dead, fifty-eight suffered from psychoses and fifteen are recorded as epileptics." About the ages of the deceased Hoffmann reported that "epilepsy kills earlier than the mental illnesses; with epilepsy most cases of death fall in the youthful period from eighteen to thirty years old, whereas the insane grow much older, and almost all deaths fall in the years from thirty to seventy."

Modern social psychiatric concepts were integrated with this focus on the natural sciences at the Frankfurt Mental Asylum. Heinrich Hoffmann supported the nonrestraint principle for free treatment, with as little coercion as possible.

Meanwhile, everyone in Frankfurt knew who Heinrich Hoffmann was. He was world renowned not so much for his scientific writings as for his children's book, *Struwwelpeter*. Under the title "Funny Stories and Comical Pictures with Fifteen Beautifully Colored Tables for Children from Three to Six Years," a picture book appeared in 1845 that later became famous. Heinrich Hoffmann hid behind the pseudonym "Reimerich Kinderlieb" and first allowed himself to be identified by his own name after the sixth edition. He had put the original manuscript, with pen-and-ink watercolor drawings, under the Christmas tree as a present for his son Carl in 1844. In 1859 Hoffmann redrew *Struwwelpeter* in a version that was translated into many languages. The stories best known to most people today are those of evil Friedrich, Little Paula with the fire, the black boy, the wild hunter, the thumb-sucker, Hans look-in-the-air, and flying Robert.[2]

The children's book author is still better known today than the psychiatrist, and as director of the city mental hospital in Frankfurt he was the first to establish a special unit for mentally ill children.

Psychoanalyst Georg Groddeck was particularly inspired by Hoffmann: "Oh Hoffmann, you wisest of all wise, people believe you made a picture book for children, but you wrote and made the song of songs of the unconscious for the grownups."[3]

In the mid-1850s Heinrich Hoffmann began intensive preparations to build a new institution on the so-called *Affenstein* (literally, "monkeystone"). The name *Affenstein* had long been common parlance, a parody of the prayer stone located there, and the hill was called the Affenstein field.

Hoffmann proved to be imaginative in procuring the necessary capital. He raised 46,000 florins through a press campaign. In addition, the Holy Spirit Hospital guaranteed a mortgage of 100,000 florins, and the Baron von Wiesenhütten promised 100,000 florins in his will.

Extensive advance work was necessary for the planning and construction of the new mental asylum, but chance also played a role. The young wife of an architect came to Hoffmann as a patient. He later related, "Well, at this time it happened that the young wife of the architect Oskar Pichler was ill with a nervous complaint. I was consulted and had her brought to the Illenau institution in Baden. The husband accompanied his sick wife and, during this otherwise unhappy time, thoroughly looked around this large institution as well as that on the Eichberg in Rheingau in the duchy of Nassau. Several weeks later he came to me and asked whether he might be able to join in the competition [for the design contract]. . . . Pichler had held most faithfully to my program. In a reasoned recommendation I pronounced myself in favor of Pichler. . . . Thus Pichler got the contract from the Office of Social Services to draw up the plans."[4]

From April 19 to July 21, 1856, the City Office of Social Services sent them both on long trips to view both old and new asylums and hospitals. Institutions throughout Europe were models for Hoffmann, so the doctor and his architect traveled via Berlin to Königsberg, to Danzig, then to Schwerin, Hamburg, Kiel, and Bremen, then through Holland and Belgium to England, where they visited the London asylum, newly constructed regional institutions, and three country asylums. They crossed France, where they toured the hospitals in Paris, Nancy, and Strassburg, and then returned to Frankfurt.

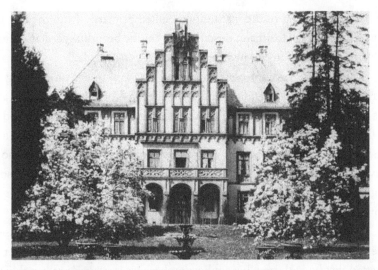

FIGURE 4.1 *The Municipal Asylum for the Insane and Epileptic in Frankfurt am Main*

It was not easy to bring the aesthetic demands of the artistically inclined architect into harmony with the practical needs of the doctor. However, they succeeded because they recognized each other as competent representatives of their respective fields and because the much-discussed question of the building style was finally decided by the city: "The institution should be constructed in the German style."

By virtue of his many visits, Hoffmann ultimately was considered an expert in asylum construction, and at the end of February 1864 he traveled to Zürich to help choose the building site for the mental institution there. At his suggestion the institution, which to this day bears this name, was built on the *Burghölzli*, the University Hospital of Psychiatry.

A few months after his trip to Zürich, in May 1864, Hoffmann moved with 100 patients into the magnificent new building, reminiscent of a fairytale castle, which the locals called the "Castle of the Insane on the Affenstein."

At first Hoffmann was the only doctor for the 100 patients, but in the fall of 1864 he received an intern, August Lotz. By 1880 the asylum was overcrowded, with 220 patients. In his memoirs he wrote, "One had to give some thought to the striking increase in the last decades of nervous illnesses, and especially the brain disorders labeled as psychoses. Humanity at present has become predominantly nervous and increasingly predisposed to nervous illnesses."

The overfilling of the institution resulted primarily from the fact that it was located, as Hoffmann described it, "in the beautiful gardens outside the city" and that "in our institution much music is made."

Even at age seventy-one, Hoffmann was still intent on running the Asylum for the Insane and the Epileptic just as before and on looking after his patients with the assistance of August Lotz. Only as he approached his eightieth year did he consider stopping. He wanted to make things a bit easier for his successor, Emil Sioli. Hoffmann thought that Sioli should have at least one colleague by his side (Lotz also intended to retire), so he obtained permission to establish an intern position and published an announcement.[5]

Many doctors, some young and inexperienced, applied in response to the announcement. A Dr. H. Kurella also applied, and Hoffmann later regretted that he withdrew his application because in 1893 Kurella published the *Naturgeschichte des Verbrechers* (*Natural History of the Criminal*) and consequently become a very well-known psychiatrist.

Thus the search for "a [class] III doctor," as interns sometimes were called at the time, dragged on. Hoffmann found the three candidates who interviewed at the asylum on March 18, 1888, unsatisfactory. The position was announced anew, and six candidates responded. But this time the applicants did not satisfy the Social Services Office for the Insane and Epileptic. The administrative director of the asylum directed a letter to the municipal authorities with the request "to announce the position again. But I would like to suggest that the fixed salary be set at 1800 marks instead of 1200 marks. The class II doctor (chief physician) receives 1500 marks and a 1000-mark personnel bonus, and in the case of a future new appointment the salary probably will not be set at less than 2500 marks. A salary of 1200 marks therefore appears too low and at any rate not enticing enough because a psychiatrist has far fewer chances of advancement than an intern at another hospital."

"And precisely with us in Frankfurt the chances of a promotion are still more limited, as in the big states, in which there are, of course, a number of regional asylums," he continued. "We therefore respectfully leave it to your discretion to empower us to advertise the position of class III doctor at 1800 marks."

The Lord Mayor's answer was unequivocal: He regarded the announcement in the *Frankfurter Zeitung* (*Frankfurt Newspaper*) and in the local gazettes as useless, saying that the position should be advertised twice each in important specialist journals, and that the word *intern*, not *class III doctor*, should be used. And, said the mayor, payment must stay at 1200 marks. The fact that the word *intern* was underlined indicates that more importance is attached to this title, which is presumably mentioned in the document for the first time, than to the designation *class III doctor*.

As a result, the following advertisement appeared in the *Deutschen Medizinal-Zeitung* (*German Medical Newspaper*), the *Berliner Klinischen Wochenschrift* (*Berlin Clinical Weekly*), the *Deutschen Medizinischen Wochenschrift* (*German Medical Weekly*), and the *Münchner Medizinischen Wochenschrift* (*Munich Medical Weekly*):

An intern is sought for the Mental Asylum at Frankfurt am Main. Salary: 1200 marks and free board and lodging. Applications requested until the end of June of this year.

Alois Alzheimer took note of this advertisement; the professional designation *intern* appealed to him more than the dubious designation *III doctor*. But before he applied an event took place that had a lasting influence on his subsequent decision to enter the field of psychiatry: He accepted a position as doctor for a mentally ill woman and traveled with her for five months. Unfortunately, who this woman was and where they traveled remain unknown.

When he returned from these travels in the fall of 1888 he took out the advertisement from the *Berliner Klinischen Wochenschrift* again and discussed it with his elder brother, Karl. They composed the application letter together but sent it off so late that it ended up bearing the date of December 14, 1888. They included a curriculum vitae in the application, as well as Alois's registration certificate, his doctoral diploma, and a recommendation from Prof. von Leube, a pioneer in the field of gastroenterological diseases, in which he certified that Alzheimer's abilities "justify great hopes."

The curriculum vitae read as follows:

The undersigned was born on June 14, 1864, at Marktbreit in Bavaria as the son of the royal judicial officer and notary Eduard Alzheimer, attended the elementary school in Marktbreit and the

*Gymnasium* in Aschaffenburg. In the fall of 1883 he began his university medical studies in Berlin and studied further at the universities of Würzburg, Tübingen, and again at Würzburg. He passed his doctoral examination in the eighth and the state examination in the ninth semester. After that he expanded his knowledge of microscopic examination methods for another semester at the Anatomical Institute with *Geheimrat* von Kölliker in Würzburg and then accepted a position as a doctor for a mentally ill woman, with whom he traveled for five months.

The brothers were sure that the passages about his accompanying a mentally ill woman as her doctor and about the "microscopic examination methods . . . at the Anatomical Institute with *Geheimrat* von Kölliker" would draw the attention of Hoffmann's successor. And that is exactly what happened. Prof. Emil Sioli was looking for someone who was both a capable doctor and a scientist who could handle a microscope.

What Alois Alzheimer and his brother could not have suspected was that the situation in Frankfurt at the end of 1888 had become dire. Hoffmann finally relinquished leadership of the clinic at age seventy-nine, as indicated by the report on the Asylum for the Insane and the Epileptic from January 1, 1888, to March 31, 1889.

Sioli succeeded Hoffmann on November 1, 1888; at the same time, medical officer Lotz, for twenty-four years Hoffmann's sole assistant, retired at full pension. Initially, a Dr. Knoblauch still served as relief doctor, but he had already accepted a position as an intern at the Heidelberg Clinic for the Insane. Therefore, Sioli stood there alone with 254 patients. Alzheimer's application seemed heaven-sent. All of Sioli's hope rested on the newly graduated Dr. Alzheimer.

Sioli did not hesitate for a moment. On the day the application arrived he promised Alzheimer the position by telegraph, although the Social Services Office had still not made its decision, and on December 19, 1888, he applied for Alzheimer's admission. The next day the Social Services Office forwarded the application to the Frankfurt municipal authorities with the request to "give Dr. Alzheimer the position; Dr. Alzheimer can start immediately." Because Dr. Sioli was completely without assistance, the Social Services Office urged the authorities "to let Dr. Alzheimer provisionally and temporarily stand in."

As emerges from the files, Alois Alzheimer was retroactively employed from December 19, 1888, on—for an annual salary of 1200 marks with a three-month period of notice. The twenty-four-year-old packed his bags in Würzburg without hesitation and set off on the most momentous journey of his life: to Frankfurt.

On the way to Frankfurt Alzheimer stopped for a night with his family in Aschaffenburg. The next day he took a coach from the main train station in Frankfurt, which brought him to Grüneburg Park, where the Municipal Asylum for the Insane and Epileptic was located.

It was not for nothing that the Asylum for the Insane and Epileptic was called the "Castle of the Insane" by the people of Frankfurt.[6] The asylum was an imposing and functionally well-planned building complex. The clinic was spacious, and there were no high walls. The front faced the city of Frankfurt and was built in the Gothic style typical of the extravagant country homes of wealthy burghers.

The rear entrance into the courtyard, with its extensive gardens, was designed like a promenade with a lane of trees. In front of the main entrance were the "gardens for paying first-class guests," the "garden for the normal class," and a garden for "the troubled patients, the paralytically ill, the epileptic, and for the raving mad." There were additional isolation gardens for the "raving mad" and a garden that belonged to the banquet hall. There were also a covered yard and a machine yard; both courtyards were located within the building.

Everything was generously laid out, with a lot of light and space, conforming to Heinrich Hoffmann's slogan, "It must above all be so that the entrance of the doctor into a unit has something of sunrise about it."[7]

## The Young Psychiatrist

In the imposing entry hall of the Frankfurt Asylum for the Insane and the Epileptic, an orderly greeted the new intern and announced him to his new boss, Prof. Emil Sioli.

Sioli's father was a landowner and had come from Solare in northern Italy. Sioli himself, twelve years older than the twenty-four-year-old Alzheimer, was from Lieskau bei Halle.[8] He had received his education in the Wietleben Asylum, where he became acquainted with early efforts to

FIGURE 4.2 *Emil Sioli*

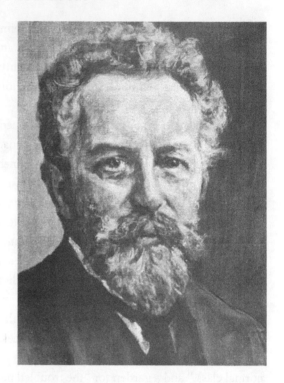

develop the most liberal possible treatment of the mentally ill in a rural setting. Like Hoffmann, Sioli held the brain to be the site of mental illness.

Sioli sincerely welcomed Alzheimer in the second-floor operating
room. The men stood facing each other: the powerfully built Alzheimer
and Sioli, an imposing figure with a full head of hair and shaggy sideburns,
a slender face, and closely set eyes.

First Sioli described the clinic to him, praising its splendid location, its
extensive parks and gardens, and the architectural beauty of the building.
A complex of pavilions, connected by covered walkways, met the latest
standards. However, the floor plan was impractical because it consisted of
rows of individual rooms—a system, said Sioli, that necessitated the use of
mechanical restraints. But, he added, there would soon be an end to that.
"The principle of open treatment," Sioli explained in one of his essays,
"demands larger rooms for the implementation of properly supervised bed
rest for those who have recently fallen ill."

Together they went back downstairs into the entrance hall, and Prof.
Sioli led Alzheimer to the framed floor plan hanging on the wall next to the

doorway. Sioli explained to Alzheimer that the similarly arranged units for women and men were subdivided into units for the quiet, the restless, the paralytic, the imbecilic, the raving, and the epileptic. He indicated to Alzheimer that they were facing a difficult time, with about 250 admissions a year and with renovation imminent.

The first days, during which young Dr. Alzheimer accustomed himself to the new work, were some of the most demanding he had ever faced. Twenty-five years later, when he had become a clinic director in Breslau, he reminisced,

> The institution accommodated only the most severely mentally ill. One had to carry out one's rounds in the restless units with powerful orderlies covering one's back, and it was sometimes necessary to fend off the attacks of irritated patients oneself. Everywhere cursing, spitting patients sat around in the corners, repulsive in their manner, peculiar in their dress, and completely inaccessible to the doctor.
>
> The most unclean habits were quite common. Some patients appeared with pockets filled with all sorts of waste, others had masses of paper and writing materials hidden all over the place and in big packets under their arms. When one had to finally follow the rules of hygiene and do something to get rid of the filth, one could not proceed without resistance and loud cries.[9]

Sioli and Alzheimer agreed that conditions could not stay this way; both believed in open treatment, were conscious of their difficult position, and were aware of the gap between demand and reality—between what they needed and what they had. Slightly embittered, Sioli wrote in his first annual report,

> If our modern principle of treatment, "nonrestraint," consisted only in the prohibition of the use of straitjackets, then we would be justified in laying claim to it; this, however, excludes coerced feeding, coerced bathing, and coerced cleaning. In that case one might as well simply build a barracks and stick a few hundred people in there. But "nonrestraint" consists in quite different things: a care for every individual patient of the kind that completely pre-

FIGURE 4.3  *Franz Nissl*

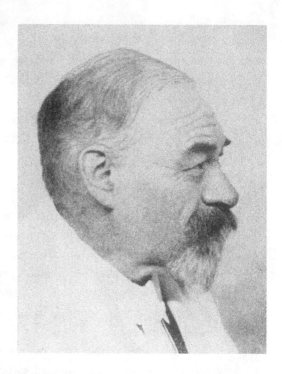

cludes the coercion attached to all of the tasks listed. It consists in keeping all stimuli away and in the most gentle, careful direction of the acute cases in more careful physical nursing, which must exceed the steps taken by other hospitals, just because they are carried out on patients who are quite seriously ill.[10]

On March 18, 1889, a senior physician finally arrived at the Frankfurt clinic: twenty-nine-year-old Dr. Franz Nissl. Nissl was a renowned physician from Munich who, before his great discovery of tissue staining, had no knowledge of microscope technique and histology. Within eight months, after numerous preliminary attempts, he found a method that soon proved groundbreaking: Nissl stain and Nissl substance (small crumbs in the nerve cells that, when one colors them with methylene blue, appear particularly vividly).

The Franconian Alzheimer and the Bavarian Nissl understood each other immediately. The two young doctors quickly formed a close friendship and met in the nearby public houses as often as the extensive duty roster allowed. Alzheimer learned from Nissl that it was the catastrophe of the Schloss Berg on Starnberg Lake that had precipitated his departure from Bavaria: The sudden death in 1886 of his medical director, Dr. Bernhard von Gudden, who drowned under mysterious circumstances together with his patient King Ludwig II, was a heavy blow for Nissl. In his curriculum vitae he wrote of it:

> On the outside everything still went on unchanged, but the all-invigorating spirit disappeared. . . . I began to lose my good health . . . and work became less and less efficient. [After a recuperative holiday and a short assignment at a Thüringen Mental Asylum,] I came to Frankfurt.[11]

Professors Sioli, Nissl, and Alzheimer were in a position to change their asylum into a progressive psychiatric hospital with the character of a sanatorium. They made their chief concern, the introduction of the nonrestraint principle, a reality and transformed the operation of the clinic from one day to the next. Alzheimer later wrote,

> All of the means of coercion, which excessive caution and nervousness in the treatment of the ill had kept in use here much longer than in most places, were cleared away in one day. In the introduction of a more intensive medical service, in the establishment of bed treatment, observation rooms, the restriction and avoidance of the use of the isolation rooms, in the establishment of duration-baths, in the guarantee to the patients of the most freedoms possible, [Sioli] went in the direction of the most progressive institutions.[12]

The institutional reorganization necessitated the further scientific education of the doctors as well as much renovation and new construction. In one of his annual reports Sioli wrote,

> The autopsy and mortuary room is currently in the middle of the building and lies in a gloomy corner of the unit for the raving mad; this is unacceptable both hygienically and aesthetically, insults the sensitivities of many patients, and makes it more difficult to complete the autopsy report. Instead of this, a separate mortu-

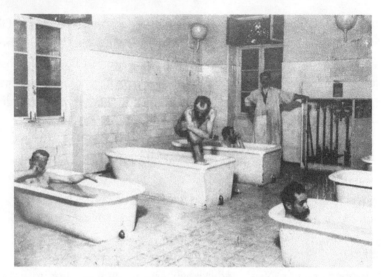

FIGURE 4.4　*Bath therapy in the Frankfurt Mental Asylum*

ary with a brightly lit autopsy room and separate morgue cellar in the rear of the institution have been applied for. Furthermore, today there is neither an actual conference or consultation room, nor a room for microscopic examinations, nor a corresponding library room.[13]

Through renovation of the existing buildings Sioli was able to introduce bed treatment in the large observation rooms. Later the duration baths were implemented as a further form of therapy, in which unruly patients could lie for hours, often for days, in a bathtub. Alzheimer was the main proponent of this method, in which the water temperature is closely regulated for the patient's comfort.[14]

Sioli, Alzheimer, and Nissl thus achieved dramatic results in treating manic and paralytic states of excitation. The bath treatment was one of their most important contributions to a biologically oriented form of psychiatric therapy.

Conversation with the patients was an important part of the treatment of mental illnesses. It demanded of the doctors an ability to win the trust of their patients and to establish a dialogue with them; they also needed the ability to listen patiently. Alzheimer and Nissl were particularly good at this and recorded many of their conversations with patients.

We still have a record of the case of the thirty-three-year-old businessman F.R., who was admitted with an atrophy of the musculature of the thumb of his left hand and the beginnings of mental illness. Alzheimer, who always performed thorough neurologic examinations, immediately recognized the muscular atrophy of the arms and twitching in the muscle fibers.

F.R. was the first patient whose case Alzheimer, together with Nissl, published.[15] On February 7, 1890, F.R. was very excited during admission, and continually screamed, "I am dead, oh, what have I done, I shot myself, I am really dead, dead, I really don't know where you are, I really don't know where I am, no, I am really in Berlin, I am really more famous than Stanley, what all have I gone through, do you know the short doctor in the public hospital, the short doctor, oh, nothing else is coming to me, you are a good doctor."

Thus it went on: uninterrupted, constantly repeated, hurried chatter. Questions thrown in between phrases remained unanswered. On February 10, 1890, Alzheimer approached F.R.'s sickbed. The patient's entire body made short, rhythmic swinging movements from left to right, approximately 120 a minute. Upon being spoken to F.R. opened his eyes and stopped moving.

Alzheimer asked, "How are you?"

The patient shook his head.

"Can't you speak?"

"Now I'm doing well again, doctor!"

"Where are you?"

The patient shook his head, breathed deeply in and out, began to rock again, and answered all further questions by shaking his head.

Alzheimer diagnosed a progressive weakening of the muscles and emaciation caused by a degeneration of the spinal marrow and the long bones, along with a diffuse disease of the nerve cells of the medulla oblongata. He meticulously documented the patient's four-week stay in a diary.

F.R. died on May 7, 1890, and Alzheimer and Nissl began the autopsy thirteen hours after his death. It confirmed Alzheimer's diagnosis: F.R. had had a progressive spinal muscle atrophy. Alzheimer saw the disease of the nerve cells of the cerebral cortex as the neuroanatomic basis of the mental disorder and published F.R.'s case in 1891.

Next to the application of the nonrestraint method and conversation therapy, the examination of organic causes of mental illnesses was the third

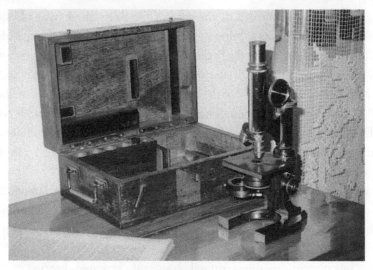

FIGURE 4.5   *Alois Alzheimer's microscope*

cornerstone of the Frankfurt clinic's success. It was made possible only by preparing and evaluating histologic slides after the autopsies.

Soon after arriving at the clinic, Alzheimer made approximately 200 slides for microscopic examination. Almost without exception they came from patients with general paresis, or paretic neurosyphilis, which, as was determined later, is a late form of syphilis. During his time in Frankfurt Alzheimer examined several hundred paretic patients and thus laid the foundation for his *Habilitation*, the postdoctoral thesis German universities require for the qualification of university lecturers.

It was fortunate for Alzheimer that two first-class researchers in the field of pathological anatomy were in Frankfurt: Carl Weigert and Ludwig Edinger.

On April 1, 1885, Weigert had become director of the Senckenberg Pathology Institute in Frankfurt. Everyone who wanted to learn the newest and best methods of histologic examination for diseased tissue had to see Weigert at the Pathology Institute. There one learned best how to "cut and stain." He is responsible for developing aniline cell nucleus stain and many other staining techniques.

Weigert completely embodied the stereotype of the absent-minded professor who gets so absorbed in a problem that he is no longer aware of his surroundings. Critics contended that he was just a "stainer" who spent too much time and effort working out technical methods.[16]

As a schoolboy of twelve Ludwig Edinger had already started to use a microscope, and from that time on he dedicated himself to science. After his studies he began to work on anatomy in a private laboratory he had constructed himself, and there he traced fiber pathways in the brain. He was the first to discover "the most important thing of all that I ever found," the previously unknown course of the pathway for the sensations of pain, temperature, and touch, the Edinger pathway.[17]

His *10 Vorlesungen über den Bau der nervösen Zentralorgane* (*Ten Lectures on the Structure of the Central Nervous Organs*) appeared in 1885. The thirty-year-old Edinger's slender volume was a creative act that for many people opened up a field that until then had been inaccessible.

As a young intern Alzheimer benefited from his direct and trusting collaboration with Franz Nissl. Nissl stain became the standard method for visualizing nerve cells; it was the basis for the cytoarchitectural examinations (to identify the cellular structure of the brain) carried out in Frankfurt.

In other words, along with Alzheimer, Nissl originated the modern histopathology of the cerebral cortex. With the help of Nissl stain Alzheimer got superb images from his microscopic slides. He did not miss an opportunity in his publications to "most enthusiastically recommend the implementation of this method everywhere, not only where the confirmation of breakdowns of fiber pathways is needed but also where proof of pathological changes in the nerve cells is important." He also made special mention of the methods developed by his friend Nissl: "For the staining of alcohol sections, dahlia, magenta red, and methylene blue in particular were used, the latter mainly with the aforementioned method developed recently by Nissl, with which one obtains quite superb images."[18]

Every medical practitioner who is familiar with these anatomic and histopathological drawings is still astounded today by the artistry with which, with the help of the camera lucida, Alzheimer made and stained his slide preparations.

With the camera lucida one can draw objects as they appear in nature. The object observed through the microscope is projected onto the drawing surface through a prism. Then one can trace the outlines of the image with a pencil and color it in.

Sioli ran the Frankfurt clinic with skill and prudence, was extremely accommodating of his co-workers, and thus stimulated their enthusiasm for work. Once a year he granted all assistant doctors a one-month working holiday, which Alzheimer called "a wonderful arrangement that makes it possible for one to concentrate again, from time to time, on scientific problems."[19]

The collegial atmosphere in the "Castle of the Insane" also fostered Alzheimer's willingness to work. He conscientiously carried out his professional duties as an intern. He was active in the sick units and persistently followed up on the cases that especially interested him outside the hours of his rounds; he examined his patients for hours, listening to them carefully, and documented their behavior.

In addition, he worked on stacks of case histories and became a very busy court-appointed expert. He was also treating a large number of private patients, without ever neglecting his beloved histologic studies. Particularly admirable in all of this was the kind calmness with which he interacted with colleagues.

Thus when Alzheimer and Nissl joined the medical staff, the Asylum for the Insane and the Epileptic began a slow but steady upswing, and the clinic's annual reports document this improvement in detail. Sioli himself prepared the reports and discussed them with Nissl and Alzheimer. They report that "more and more use is made of the baths; apart from regular monthly cleaning baths for all patients, ninety-two female and eighty-seven male patients receive protracted medicinal baths lasting from a half an hour to an hour, sometimes for weeks, sometimes for months. Forty-eight male and thirty-two female patients receive therapeutic mud wraps of several hours' duration, also for weeks on end."[20]

Meanwhile, the treatment had "become completely free. Means of coercion are no longer used, narcotic medicines are used sparingly. Usually, paraldehyde is given, on average, fourteen individual doses per day of 3 to 6 grams, more rarely Sulfonal, and still less often chloral." Morphine injections were used in certain indicated cases: "This, along with wrappings, proves useful in treating the severely agitated and the paretic. In the treatment of the most seriously ill, bedridden, and those with a tendency to uncleanliness and bedsores, wood-fiber beds appear to be most appropriate for most cases. . . . The institution covers around 37 acres, and alongside the large park there are extensive vegetable gardens, so that 30 percent of the patients are also successfully occupied in the park and with gardening. A tailor's shop and a bookbindery have been established as workshops next to the existent carpenter's workshop. In winter, woodcutting and straw-weaving are the main activities."

Smaller excursions were offered from the asylum into nearby areas. The reports describe "a big excursion with 120 patients to the beautiful Königstein and Eppstein, together with climbing the castle," and a series of concert evenings in the asylum, performances of short comedies by the participants, and even a summer festival with music and dance. At the concert evenings both the doctors and the patients enjoyed the efforts of their own mixed choir and vociferously honored the cooperation of well-known Frankfurt artists who made their skills in singing, instrumental music, and oratory available for a good cause.

Frankfurt's residents, initially very skeptical about the new methods Heinrich Hoffmann's successors had introduced, started to trust the young doctors in the "Castle of the Insane." Meanwhile, scientific colleagues began to pay attention to the address on the Affenstein.

## Recognition in the Scientific World

"After the considerations expressed in the discussion regarding the practicability of treating states of excitement with protracted baths, I have to mention that at the Frankfurt Asylum this method has not proven difficult to implement at all and has proven itself highly useful."[21]

Long, continuous knocking on the lecture hall benches—the German academic manner of applause—followed these closing words from the twenty-eight-year-old Dr. Alzheimer. In a well-structured lecture at the 1892 Karlsruhe Conference of Southwest German Psychiatrists he had reported on the terrible conditions he had discovered in 1888 in Frankfurt in the restless patient units: Patients, undressed and chilled through, lay on torn straw sacks and mattresses in cells smeared with food remains and feces.

Alzheimer had told how he, together with Hoffmann's successor as clinic director, Prof. Sioli, soon introduced the bathing treatment, "with which conditions changed abruptly. The introduction of permanent bathing proved to be an uncommonly beneficial practice."

Alzheimer's lecture and discussion contributions strongly supported the argument of psychiatrist Emil Kraepelin, already a well-known and influential figure. In 1891 Kraepelin had spoken, also in Karlsruhe, on positive experiences with duration bathing and made a statement on keeping the water temperature constant: "The water temperature is continually monitored by personnel and regulated as much as possible according to the comfort of the patients through the addition of warm or cold water; it fluctuates a little around 34 degrees Celsius."[22]

In light of Alzheimer's lecture, Kraepelin and Sioli were very excited about the positive experiences with the duration bath treatment, especially with manic and paretic states of agitation: "All means of coercion still in use, such as tight gloves, indestructible suits, and, above all, isolation, are made almost completely unnecessary."

Clearly the Karlsruhe Congress impressed itself particularly strongly on Kraepelin's memory; he later remarked in his memoirs that to his astonishment his duration bath therapy initially encountered intense resistance. However, it was supported by several other psychiatrists, particularly by Alzheimer, "who had seen our arrangements and implemented them in Frankfurt."[23]

The triumvirate of Sioli, Nissl, and Alzheimer gradually made a name for itself at the scientific congresses. The three presented brilliant lectures and contributed, through intelligent discussion remarks, to the progress of their young science. One of Alzheimer's lectures made a special impression during the meeting of the Association of German Psychiatrists that took place in Dresden from September 21 to 22, 1894.

Eighty-five prominent psychiatrists participated. The meeting began by commemorating the deceased Dr. Lotz of Frankfurt, who had stood at Heinrich Hoffmann's side for so many years.

Then Alzheimer spoke. He gave an account of the progress of his research and lectures on what had become his favorite topic, arteriosclerosis of the brain. He drew special attention by emphasizing microscopic findings in the brain that allowed recognition of the changes in the brain vessels down into the smallest branches. He said that he had observed twelve patients and that in none of them—in contrast to patients with general paresis—could syphilis be shown to be the cause of their symptoms.

Alzheimer emphasized that arteriosclerotic brain atrophy was not only clinically but also anatomically distinct from general paresis, with which it had previously been classified. The essential distinguishing feature was the more focal character of arteriosclerotic degeneration, in contrast to diffuse paretic changes.

With that finding, Alzheimer pointed to the future. Almost a hundred years later physicians identified multi-infarct dementia, the loss of early-acquired intellectual abilities through numerous small brain infarctions, that is, occlusions or transpositions of the smallest arteries in the brain and the brain stem.

Sioli supported Alzheimer in discussion: "I believe that patients may come less often to the mental asylum because the dementia is different: The memory lapses are predominant, and there are no personality defects. I often found attacks of cardiophobia [an irrational fear of heart disease] with a pronounced awareness of the illness."

Moeli, director of a recently constructed clinic in Berlin-Lichtenberg, highlighted dementia still more: "I see in this group of illnesses more a form of senile brain transformations. High-grade amnesia and the peculiar state of confusion move it decisively closer to senile dementia."

Then Emil Kraepelin, somewhat skeptical and keen on trick questions, turned to Alzheimer: "My colleague Alzheimer, could you exclude traumas as causes?"

And when Jolly, the Berlin *Ordinarius* (Full Professor) of Psychiatry, confirmed, "I am also convinced that Alzheimer's cases are close to dementia senilis, and I'd go so far as to interpret arteriosclerotic dementia as an early form of dementia senilis," the questions and comments flowed.

Alzheimer responded first to Kraepelin: "I could exclude traumas, diabetes, nephritis, and an uncompensated heart insufficiency." To Moeli and Jolly he replied, "I too am of the view that my cases are very close to dementia senilis and that it would be a mistake to classify them with general paresis. But I can sharply distinguish them from so-called dementia senilis praecox."[24]

This was a remarkable statement because seven years later the unequivocal distinction between senile and presenile dementia led, during the examination of Auguste D., to the emergence of one of the most important names in medicine: *Alzheimer's disease.*

The president opened the second day of the annual meeting of the Association of German Psychiatrists in Dresden, September 22, 1894, with deep seriousness: "Gentlemen, I ask you to stand up from your seats. I have the sad duty to inform you that our highly esteemed colleague, Medical Consul Dr. Heinrich Hoffmann, former director of the Frankfurt Mental Asylum, died yesterday at the age of eighty-five."[25] The warmly felt words with which the president honored Hoffmann moved the congress participants deeply. Afterwards, Prof. Mendel from Berlin spoke on "The Mentally Ill in the Draft of the Civil Code for the German Reich After the Second Reading." The record of the session notes,

> The speaker begins with a reference to his discussion of this question at the annual meeting of the Association of German Psychiatrists at Bonn in 1888. Now, he says, that the second reading of the draft is so fully supported by the *Reichscommission* that a resolution has already been passed on the essential points that at that time prompted consideration, it appears, according to the speaker, time to relay the results.

What followed were explanations of "the possibility of being able to declare habitual drinkers, who become dangers to themselves or others or are unable to act on their own behalf, incapable of managing their own affairs." Mendel then read out the version chosen by the *Reichscommission* on the possibilities of declaring someone incapacitated:

> Incapacitation takes place
>     1. due to mental illness, when the mentally ill person as a consequence thereof is not able to take care of his affairs,
>     2. due to wastefulness,
>     3. due to alcoholism, when the drinker as a consequence thereof is not able to take care of his obligations or exposes himself or his family to the danger of a state of emergency or threatens the security of others.

On legal incompetence Mendel reported that the commission, in agreement with his recommendation, drafted the regulation in the following way:

78. Legally incompetent is one who finds himself in a condition of pathological disturbance of mental functioning, through which his free exercise of will is precluded.

79. The declaration of the intent of a legally incompetent person is null and void. Void also is the declaration of intent that is given in a condition of unconsciousness of the exclusion of the free determination of intent.

Mendel reported further that, at his suggestion, the commission extended 79 to include the mental illnesses of spouses:

A spouse can sue for divorce when the other spouse has succumbed to mental illness, the illness has lasted three years during the marriage and has reached a degree that precludes spiritual companionship, and the prospect of reestablishing the companionship is precluded.

Then Mendel elaborated on cases in which criminal acts are committed under the influence of alcohol or other drugs, a question that was of particular interest to Alzheimer as a forensic psychiatrist. The session record continues,

The paragraph that fixes responsibility for the harm one inflicts on another when the use of reason is impaired by self-induced drunkenness—in contrast to the cases where a loss of the use of reason through other causes exists—has taken a form in the commission that can be described as substantially better and as at least somewhat taking into account the psychiatric considerations raised. It now runs,

"§750. A person is not responsible for harm inflicted on another in a condition of unconsciousness or in a condition of diseased disorder of mental activity that impairs the free determination of intention. If someone has put himself into temporary condition of this kind through alcoholic beverages or similar means, then he is responsible for any unlawfully caused damage in the same way as if he were responsible for negligence, unless he fell into that state without fault."

This version corresponded to the concerns the psychiatrists had previously raised. The following resolution was passed unanimously:

> The Association of German Psychiatrists expresses its satisfaction that the resolutions of the second reading of the civil code substantially fulfill the requirements that the association set forth with reference to the relationship of the mentally ill to the determinations of the civil code.

The civil code (*Das Bürgerliche Gesetzbuch*, or BGB) came into effect in 1900.

Alzheimer and Sioli had congress fever and immediately traveled from Dresden to Vienna, where German natural scientists were holding their sixty-sixth meeting from September 24 to 30.

Privy Councillor Richard, Baron von Krafft-Ebing, the director of the Second Psychiatric Clinic in Vienna, opened the meeting. Krafft-Ebing was well known in his field as the author of two important works, *Das Lehrbuch der Psychiatrie* (*The Textbook of Psychiatry*) and *Psychopathia sexualis*.

In Vienna Alzheimer spoke on a topic with which he had been engaged since the beginning of his clinical training: general paresis in children, adolescents, and young adults, the "*paralysis progressiva* of the developmental years."[26] He distinguished the early form of paresis, with reference to the causes of illness, the anatomy, and the course of the disease, from paresis in adults. Alzheimer knew how to engage his audience after a necessarily dry introduction: "Three cases that I have examined concern young girls." He then briefly described the particulars of the cases, also giving details of the parents' histories, especially those of the fathers.

> Gentlemen, I want to present you with an exemplary case. It concerns an young girl born illegitimately. The mother was a prostitute, often convicted, syphilitic, and probably also suffering from general paresis. The father was also previously convicted and— gentlemen, let me put it this way—dissipated "*in Baccho et Venere*."
>
> At age twenty-one the young woman herself observed a decline in her ability to see and was admitted to the hospital. There

examination found an atrophy of the optic nerves, headaches, shooting pains in the back, and the absence of a patellar reflex.

At age twenty-six the patient was admitted to our asylum with states of agitation. She showed typical symptoms such as fibrillary twitching of the tongue and facial musculature, high-grade dementia, paralytic attacks, temporary states of agitation, and megalomania.

I saw the patient, a maid, A.F., for myself on July 19, 1894, because of "fits of rage" and asked,

"Were you always blind?"

"Yes."

"Could you see before?"

"Yes."

"Since when have you been unable to see?"

"Four, five years ago."

"What year is it now?"

"1889."

"Month?"

"I don't know."

"Summer?"

"Yes."

"Or winter?"

"Yes."

"4 × 5?"

"20." She laughs.

"6 × 7?"

"20."

"How are you?"

"Good."

"Are you happy?"

She laughs.

"How long have you been here?"

She laughs.

"Where are you?"

"Dieburg."

In Dieburg, gentlemen, there she was still a young innocent girl, before she went to the city! Then I asked her,

"Who am I?"

She laughs.

"How old are you?"

"Twenty-two."

"Born when?"

"1867."

"What amuses you so?"

She laughs.

"Are you blind?"

"Yes."

"But isn't that very sad?"

She laughs.

"Do you have pains?"

She laughs.

So much for the maid A.F., gentlemen. I thoroughly examined all three cases in the same way. One case was so complicated that I had to call in Ludwig Edinger as a neurologic consultant for advice.

Our colleagues who referred us the cases clearly had difficulties in making a precise diagnosis because the behavior of the three girls was misleading. And so it happened that a series of specialists who had observed the patients had made the diagnoses of brain tumor, multiple sclerosis, and lues of the central nervous system, whereas nobody thought of juvenile paresis.

Alzheimer concluded his description of the case of A.F.'s illness with the words, "It saddens me, gentlemen, that only the autopsy can finally bring clarity."

The publication of the cases appeared in 1896.[27] Alzheimer could then show that juvenile paresis manifested itself predominantly between the thirteenth and sixteenth years. On average it lasted just under five years, longer than paresis in adults. Both sexes were equally afflicted among juveniles, in contrast to adults, among whom patients were predominantly male. Otherwise, Alzheimer could uncover no fundamental differences between juvenile paresis and the adult form and saw no reason to distinguish a particular clinical form of paresis in the adolescent years.

## First Publications

"A Born Criminal," an especially well-executed essay by Alois Alzheimer, appeared in 1896 in the *Archiv der Psychiatrie und Nervenkrankheiten* (*Archive of Psychiatry and Nervous Illnesses*).[28] It is entertainingly and excitingly written and offers insight into Alzheimer's practice as a forensic physician.

He describes the case of Oskar M., who was admitted to the mental asylum in Frankfurt on March 16, 1894, and stayed there for six weeks, where he was treated by Alzheimer. Dr. H. Kurella had written his book on the natural history of the criminal. He also had something to say about Oskar M.:

> In this case we are dealing with a swindler who, like the "pill-scrounging" (epilepsy-simulating) vagrants of the fifteenth century, pretends to have an interesting nervous illness to live from deceit . . . and who could deceive a really smart teacher of psychiatry.

Oskar M. was a young theology student who repeatedly attracted attention through begging, trickery, and embezzlement and who kept the psychiatrists, public prosecutors, and courts constantly busy. As with all research subjects, Alzheimer performed the clinical examinations himself and made inquiries about all information that could possibly indicate a pathological disposition in the family, "to place our renewed appraisal on the broadest foundation and thereby to elucidate the reasons that led to contradictory assessments of O. in the reports of Kurella and the other experts."

Remarkably, he also carefully measured sections of Oskar M.'s skull, which revealed striking asymmetries in the face and other parts of the head. Thus Alzheimer found that the right ear, at 7 centimeters, was noticeably longer than the left, at 6.5 centimeters. He found a narrower palpebral fissure on the right than on the left, whereby the nose ran from the right at the top to the left at the bottom. Alzheimer put a great deal of effort into clearing up this case, and he succeeded in tracking down a fetishist:

> Because our knowledge of . . . [his] sexual feelings came only from O.'s statements, I wanted to make an effort to determine more closely the degree of their reliability through objective observation.

On April 9, I unobtrusively left female footwear of the kind that O. claimed tended especially to arouse him in the chief guard's wardrobe, which I had allocated to O. for his writing. I instructed the chief guard, as was otherwise often the case, to occupy himself with something else, to stay there, and to continue to keep an eye on O.'s behavior.

O. was writing in the middle of the room, and the chief guard reported that O. was remarkable only in his increased restlessness and that he often looked toward the footwear. When, after a brief absence, the guard reentered the room, he found O. occupied with the shoes, touching them and examining them closely. I could see that on this particular day O. did not get as far along with his work as he otherwise tended to.

In the evening he appeared somewhat restless and had a gloomy facial expression. When I asked about his health, he claimed to feel well. His pulse, which I had repeatedly taken and found constantly between 80 and 85 beats per minute, was at 125 beats.

When I urged him the next day to finish his work soon, he told me that he had been unable to work properly in the last few days and claimed, after further inquiries, that the reason was that he had been so excited by the view of the ladies' shoes in the chief guard's room that he had found it difficult to collect his thoughts. His pulse remained over 120.

In the following days he appeared somewhat depressed, and I once established a pulse of 65 beats a minute. Several days later he displayed his normal behavior again and his pulse was once again continuously around 80 beats.

Alzheimer concluded that Oskar M. had a hereditary degenerative mental disorder. He saw Oskar M.'s sexual fetish as its most striking symptom and sharply criticized previous experts who had not ascribed any meaning to the important signs of anatomic degeneration. As occurred so often in such cases, the previous experts had held completely different views and described Oskar M. as an "incorrigible crook" and a "congenital candidate for a mental asylum."

When Alzheimer was called to give an expert opinion on Oskar M. in court, he contested the existence of signs of degeneration that were supposed to be "peculiar to the criminal or the insane alone." He expressly emphasized that research had not yet succeeded in identifying unequivocal signs of degeneration that would make it possible to distinguish criminals from the mentally ill.

Later, in his reminiscences of *25 Years of Psychiatry*, Alzheimer described just how difficult it was at that time for a psychiatrist to be convincing before the court:

> The relationship of psychiatry to the administration of justice has changed substantially. If one was called to court as an expert—this happened in those days far less often than it does today—then one did not have an easy relationship with the judges and public prosecutors. A mutual understanding between the two world views often appeared impossible.
>
> The basis of the judge's thought and action is formed by the deductive concepts of his jurisprudence, the psychiatrist's by scientific observation and experience. The judge demands expiation, the psychiatrist simply protection and defense of society from harm. It was not at all rare for one to hear unfounded mistrust between the lines of the public prosecutor's pronouncements: the notions that the psychiatrist holds every person to be ill and that if one wants to wrench the accused from the arms of justice, all forms of justice would therefore have to suffer. For this reason, too, psychiatric suggestions for reform could hardly encounter understanding.

In the case of Oskar M., Alzheimer explained the clinical picture entirely in the terms of modern forensic psychiatry and ascribed the serious inhibitions of bone growth development in Oskar M.'s skull to a hereditary condition.

Alzheimer found pathogenic signs of degeneration and accompanying brain development disorders with corresponding psychological peculiarities, which were important before the court in Oskar M.'s case. In his closing plea Alzheimer put things clearly and unmistakably:

> We hold that Oskar M. suffers from a hereditary degenerative mental disorder. The most conspicuous sign of his illness is a sex-

ual perversity in the form of fetishism. It manifests with all the
signs of an obsession and a compulsive act and does so with an unmistakable periodicity. The vagabond-like way of life and O.'s
swindling are consequences of the same. In addition, O. shows the
character anomalies of many hereditary mental degenerates.

Unmistakable in Alzheimer's plea is familiarity with Cesar Lombroso's famous study of the "*uomo delinquente.*"[29] According to Lombroso,
born criminals were people who, on the basis of a formative deficiency,
were stuck at an earlier level of development and therefore in their physical and mental characteristics resembled people of past cultural epochs.

Alzheimer rejected this theory decisively. As he wrote elsewhere, the
predispositions of violent criminals were not, as Lombroso had represented them, to be traced back to "atavism" and regression to an earlier cultural stage "but rather [to be sought] for the most part in a pathological pecu-
liarity of the mental condition, in a diseased psychological degeneration";
he thus declared himself unequivocally in favor of the degeneration theory
of Bénédict Morel.

In his main work on physical and moral degeneration, *Traité des
dégénérescences physiques et morales humaines* (*Treatise on Human Physical
and Moral Degeneration*), Morel postulated a "degeneration" that increases
across generations through dubious ways of life. In the first generation,
Morel said, this can be observed in a nervous temperament, moral incompetence, and dissipation; in the second in an inclination to serious neurosis;
in the third in psychological disorders, suicide, and mental incompetence;
and in the fourth via congenital imbecility, deformities, and developmental
deficiencies. According to Morel, if children of this generation reach pu-
berty, they develop the disease of decay, which Morel called dementia
praecox, a psychosis with a rapid outcome of stupor.

By virtue of his detailed investigation of physical traits—as in the
case of Oskar M.—Alzheimer demonstrated early in his tenure as a senior physician his mastery of both neurology and psychiatry. This is one
reason why Kraepelin later nominated him as editor of the *Zeitschrift für
die Gesamte Neurologie und Psychiatrie* (*Journal of Complete Neurology and
Psychiatry*).

Alzheimer devoted increasing attention to the pathological anatomy of
the cerebral cortex and the anatomic foundations of psychoses. Inex-

haustible, he also paid close attention to his recently admitted patients and made records of interviews with them as chief physician.

Given the "extraordinary confusion that dominates in psychiatric nomenclature," he knew that it was important "to produce detailed case histories that do not force the reader to believe in the correctness of his diagnosis but rather make it possible for him to form a clinical judgment for himself." It sounded almost prophetic when he remarked to Nissl, "But the former master builder will be able to use them purposefully only when he can also examine the clinical images of the individual cases with his own eyes and evaluate them for himself."[30]

In 1895 Alzheimer published an article that drew on his daily clinical work.[31] In it he related how he had produced optic illusions in five patients with epileptic psychosis and paralysis through pressure on the eyeball, thus proving that "this sensory illusion, which everyone can reproduce in himself in a clinically insignificant form," is not, as had previously been assumed, "specific to the delirium of the alcoholic" but rather could also be produced in patients with other psychiatric symptoms such as madness, epileptic and hysterical psychoses, and general paresis.

He could thereby show that the pressure-induced hallucinations did not rest on the power of suggestion. Even with the use of the most suggestive questions, the visions could not be triggered in other patients who were no less susceptible to suggestion. Shortly before this, Alzheimer had become acquainted with the so-called Liepmann experiment, in which these "pressure-visions" could be produced and in which the sun, moon, clouds, sky, stars, or entire scenes could be seen; particularly frequently, the illusion of written and printed things could be produced.

On March 7, 1896, a sixty-two-year-old married bookkeeper, P.D., was brought to the asylum. A week later, on March 14, Alzheimer went to see him.

The patient cowered in a corner of the isolation room, chamber pot in hand, and fearfully asked over and over again, "What's supposed, what I am supposed then, so what do they want there?"

He let Alzheimer put him to bed but repeated again and again, "But I can't die like this."

A little later he became somewhat calmer and clearer; Alzheimer began again with his typical questions:

"Where are you?"

"The mental institution or something, but I don't actually know where it was."

"How long have you been here?"

"A few minutes."

"Where were you before?"

"I don't know, I don't know, mental asylum or where I was."

"Why here?"

"Because I couldn't state where I am from and what I am."

"What year is it?"

"96."

"Which month?"

"That I cannot state."

Alzheimer insisted on an answer: "Approximately?"

"I wanted before, I don't know anymore, I wanted to speak to Dr. B., in the literary institution. I was released there, I believe, but I quite certainly would still like to speak to Dr. B., the last time I said, everything is by the book. I don't know what will happen in the future, because I have the result yesterday, I didn't sign anything in the house, I'm just heading to the commotion, now the guy is gone, I didn't sign any more, I can't sign any more, oh God, oh God, what still goes on!"

Alzheimer asked, "Are you frightened that something will happen to you?"

"Yes, if I don't sign, I can't go, yesterday he already wanted to kill me, the one who brought the keys, but he is gone, I'm afraid, someone wants to, the wounds, burn me. He doesn't even have a subpoena, he always asked me what I wanted, he always had the first sign, he also handed the air cushion over to me, Dr. B. can confirm it."

Just as thoroughly as with the bookkeeper, P.D., Alzheimer examined the businessman's seventeen-year-old daughter M.S. and the thirty-two-year-old seamstress M.D.

Alzheimer classified these three cases among the so-called exhaustion psychoses. Later examination of the slide preparations made from these patients' brains after death showed how closely these three cases resembled each other.

In 1897 he published the results of his research under the title "Contributions to the Pathological Anatomy of the Cerebral Cortex and to the Anatomic Basis of Some Psychoses" in the *Monatsschrift für Neurologie und*

*Psychologie* (*Monthly Journal of Neurology and Psychology*).[32] In all three cases he described extensive pathological changes in the nerve cells in all cortical layers, with extensive inconspicuous stroma and connective tissue. The changes were so alike that it was hardly possible "to distinguish a section from the first case from one from the second and third cases."

He nevertheless warned against assuming an anatomic basis for the exhaustion psychoses based on the changes he described, stressing that in the majority of clinical pictures of psychotic conditions no anatomic bases existed at all, quite in contrast to symptoms in internal medicine, for example, where anatomic causes had already been well known for a long time and individual diseases had already been described.

Alzheimer also warned against examining pathological changes in the cerebral cortex with inadequate methods because such work would only "impede the progress of our knowledge of the anatomy of the psychoses."

Careful and self-critical as ever, in evaluating these three cases Alzheimer concluded that he "merely has several building blocks in hand" to which "still many others have to be added, until they can form a building."

The Frankfurt clinic also treated epileptics. At the time, there was no conclusive knowledge about the anatomic basis of epilepsy and epileptic stupor.

With two patients, whom he examined painstakingly, Alzheimer succeeded in showing anatomic changes by performing autopsies and subjecting their brains to histopathological examination.

The first patient, Theodor H., was thirty-two years old and the son of a gardener. Alzheimer went up to his bed and asked him,

"What is your name?"

"H."

"How old are you?"

"Thirty-two years."

"What day is it today?"

"Wednesday." (*wrong answer*)

"Month?"

"November."

"Year?"

"1861."

"In which year were you born?"

"1861."

H. counted fingers held up before him incorrectly but made few errors in arithmetic:

"2 × 2?"

"4."

"4 × 8?"

"32."

"9 + 7?"

"16."

"Where are you?"

"In a butcher shop."

"What kind of a room is that?"

"The wall, 3 × 2 = 5."

H. saw an inkwell, reached for it, and named it correctly. He recognized a fountain pen from a distance of 1 meter and a handkerchief from a distance of 2 meters. He correctly identified a 1-mark piece, but a 10-mark piece he called a 1-mark piece. He made an unsteady hand movement in reaching for it. To Alzheimer's question about convulsions he replied, "When twice a day probably—very bad—long—out of it."

Alzheimer also described H.'s convulsive states:

If one observes him longer, one notes that his movements, obviously caused by ideation, are accompanied by involuntary convulsive movements of the head and arms; at times the movements that travel across them are sudden, and at times they seem forced, and the head and arms spin out. The movements appear disorderly and flailing upon preliminary observation. A complicated convulsive movement in which the arm, drawn in at the elbow, travels until it reaches overhead to the nape of the neck recurs especially frequently.

To the many questions directed at him, H. answered merely, "Where is my brother—the two things at the register." Then the jerky, convulsive movements recurred over and over, followed by a convulsive tonic state that gripped his entire body for several seconds with apparent loss of consciousness.

Then, suddenly, H. called out to the ceiling, "Shut your mouth up there, you common pigdog!" He then threatened with his hands toward the

ceiling and screamed, "Who is up there?—my sister—is she telling someone off?—1861."

In May 1897 the frequency of the attacks increased. In the last days before death the attacks occurred so frequently that they could no longer be
counted; between attacks, a dazed state predominated. The patient finally
died of pneumonia.

The second case concerned Katharina Anna K., a forty-year-old patient. After the onset of attacks she became increasingly irritable and intolerable, threatening her husband and children with a knife, throwing burning lamps around, and incorrectly performing simple household tasks. One
day she poured coffee grounds over a cooked, ready-to-serve pot roast.
The microscopic findings on postmortem brain examination resembled
those of Theodor H.

Alzheimer published his investigations in 1898, again in the *Monatsschrift für Neurologie und Psychiatrie* (*Monthly Journal of Neurology and Psychiatry*), under the title "A Contribution to the Pathological Anatomy of
Epilepsy."[33] He summarized his results as follows:

> 1. There are cases of so-called genuine, that is, congenital
> epilepsy, in which characteristic pathological-anatomic changes
> appear. Macroscopically, one sees a wrinkled, finely bumpy sur-
> face on the gyri and a more or less clear sclerosis of the surface lev-
> el of the cortex. What makes an impression microscopically is an
> increase of glia [stroma and nutrient tissue of the nervous system
> between the nerve cells and blood vessels], with the striking ten-
> dency to fit into the normal formation of the glia, and a consider-
> able loss of marrow-containing fibers and nerve cells in the cere-
> bral cortex. The degeneration is spread over the entire cerebral
> cortex.
>
> 2. Many findings suggest that the nervous substance is prima-
> rily diseased, and
>
> 3. The histologic changes explain epileptic dementia.

Alzheimer thus successfully connected neurologic symptoms and psychological phenomena with a disease of the brain.

In 1898 Alzheimer published extensively on senile dementia, which develops in a phase of life "where the brain has, on average, already under-

gone a serious loss of weight, and regular signs of a senescence, a premature aging, can be shown," and on brain diseases with a basis in arteriosclerosis. He thereby grasped for the first time a series of questions that later did not become the focal point of his research but made him world-famous.

In the *Monatsschrift für Neurologie und Psychiatrie* Alzheimer published "Recent Work on Dementia Senilis,"[34] which includes a passage indicating that in Frankfurt in the early 1890s he had already seen a patient who, though still young, had become zombie-like and therefore was classified as "presenile demented":

> But then I examined a case that could be described as presenile de-
> mentia and in which seriously atrophied processes appeared on the
> nerve cells but were accompanied by insignificant atheromatous
> vascular changes. This case permits the assumption that, apart
> perhaps from nutritional disturbances, which cause vascular dis-
> ease, a congenitally inherited weakness of the central nervous sys-
> tem could also have premature atrophy of the ganglial cells as a
> consequence. Admittedly, degenerative changes of the ganglial
> cells that are independent of vascular disease could also occur in
> typical cases of dementia senilis.

But Alzheimer, always cautious in his conclusions, remarked immedi- ately that "naturally this case too still does not appear conclusive, and fur- ther investigations are still needed to strengthen the above assumptions." It is therefore understandable why three years later, on November 26, 1901, Alzheimer took such intense interest in Auguste D.: She was the decisive piece in the dementia puzzle.

In the same publication Otto Binswanger was mentioned for the first time. Alzheimer devoted an entire paragraph to what became known as Bin- swanger's disease, a subcortical arteriosclerotic encephalopathy—a microan- giopathy of the brain—in which the smallest vessels become diseased:

> Furthermore, a certain special place is due to imbecility in the
> aged, dementia praesenilis, to which Binswanger has devoted a
> brief account. According to Binswanger, it strikes people whose
> mental development from adolescence on had been meager but
> whose weaknesses in judgment from the end of their forties on al-

ready show a broader and increasing loss. They become slow, dull, and indifferent, and their memories show appreciable gaps. Physically too they appear more worn out, speech and movement are trembling and shaky. Easily excited, they overestimate their abilities and perform imprudent actions, which often lead to their institutionalization.

Presenile dementia distinguishes itself from the usual senile dementia through the preexisting mental weaknesses and the early occurrence of senile insanity and distinguishes itself from general paresis through its long period of stagnation, as well as through the lack of the physical characteristics of general paresis.

In further publications Alzheimer chose topics that barely overlapped with each other. He thus qualified himself early on as an extremely versatile psychiatrist, one who not only published observations drawn from daily clinical practice but also addressed contemporary questions with ramifications for social medical problems. He generally published his work in the *Zentralblatt für Nervenheilkunde und Psychiatrie* (*Central Paper of Neurology and Psychiatry*).

Furthermore, alongside his numerous publications Alzheimer spoke at the most important congresses; in fact, his activity at congresses increased toward the end of the century.

In September 1895 the Association of German Psychiatrists convened in Hamburg, where Alzheimer presented microscopic slide preparations of two typical cases of brain degeneration.

In 1896 the Assembly of German Scientists and Doctors convened in Frankfurt. Alzheimer gave a lecture on "The Anatomic Spread of Processes of Paretic Degeneration."

Also in 1896 the Association of German Psychiatrists held its annual convention in Heidelberg. Alzheimer gave an account of five cases of a severe arteriosclerosis. Some of the congress participants, including Alzheimer, congregated again in the clinic on the Sunday morning, where Kraepelin presented a series of patients with motor disorders and in varying states of health, and then discussed the cases extensively with their colleagues.

In 1897 the Southwest German Neurologists and Psychiatrists convened in Baden-Baden under the auspices of their twenty-second Traveling Conference. Alzheimer talked about acute delirium and illustrated his lecture with photographs.

The conference of Southwest German Psychiatrists took place in November 1898 in Heidelberg. Alzheimer gave an account—again with many micrographs—of the pathological anatomy of mental disorders in extreme old age. The director of the Frankfurt Clinic, Prof. Sioli, invited the assembly to Frankfurt for the next year. The invitation was accepted—a great honor for the clinic and its doctors.

In Frankfurt, clinical lectures on individual groups of mental disorders were held in the asylum, and they were attended by many doctors from the city and environs. The 1899 report notes, "Last winter these lectures were classified as part of the continuing education course for local doctors in the city. . . . Other courses that took place included the irregular continuing medical education course for doctors from out of town and a three-week lecture series on acute psychosis by Dr. Alzheimer."

Concerning the further development of the Asylum for the Insane and Epileptic toward the end of the nineteenth century, it was reported,

> In recent years there have been four salaried doctors apart from the director active in the asylum, so that there was one salaried doctor for every eighty-five continuing patients. . . .
>
> On December 28, 1898, the intern Dr. Lilienstein left after nine months of industrious work in the service of the asylum to specialize in nervous illnesses at Bad Nauheim. Dr. Julius Raecke took over his position but then left after a year and seven months to take an intern position at the University Clinic for the Insane in Tübingen. He was followed by Dr. Korbinian Brodmann. Since February 1, 1899, Dr. Adolf Friedländer has occupied a trainee position at the asylum.[35]

That Frankfurt at that time was a talent forge for psychiatry is proven by the further careers of three of the doctors named in the report. Raecke later became a professor of psychiatry in Frankfurt, and Brodmann became director of the topographic–histologic unit of the German Research Institute for Psychiatry in Munich. Several cytoarchitectural fields in the human cerebral cortex are named after him.

Friedländer, who had moved from the Senckenberg Institute to psychiatry, remained with Sioli for four years. He later acquired a large property in Taunus for construction of the Private Clinic *Hohe Mark* in Taunus, which became popular among German and foreign high nobility. Until World War I, patients of high rank and standing could occupy entire houses with their domestic staff there.

Yet before the construction of his imposing clinic, which in many respects resembled the "Castle of the Insane," Friedländer examined countless patients under Alzheimer's direction, including Auguste D.

## Years of Happiness

In 1892 a telegram reached Alzheimer from Algeria. It had been sent by Wilhelm Erb, a famous neurologist from Heidelberg, after whom Erb–Charcot disease, Duchenne–Erb paralysis, and other conditions are named. Erb urgently needed the help of his colleague and friend just when Sioli, Nissl, and Alzheimer had their hands full looking after their patients, supervising renovations, and conducting research in the microscopy room late in the night.

For a long time Erb had been treating Otto Geisenheimer, a diamond dealer, who was suffering from a general paresis popularly called softening of the brain. After undergoing a successful treatment in Heidelberg, Geisenheimer had invited Erb to accompany him as his personal physician on a scientific expedition to north Africa. Geisenheimer brought along his wife, Cecilie Simonette Nathalie.

The expedition party had barely reached north Africa when Geisenheimer, who also suffered from neurasthenia, had a nervous breakdown. Erb recalled the medical and psychiatric skills of Alois Alzheimer, who, years ago, had told him about his five-month trip with the mentally ill woman.

Alzheimer was the recognized specialist on the clinical picture of general paresis: He had already published on its early form, and he was the only one who could successfully treat both adults and children. The latter quality was especially important because Geisenheimer's daughter, Marion, also needed treatment. So Erb requested that Alzheimer come to Algeria immediately to treat the prominent patient on the spot and, if need be, bring him, with his wife, back to Germany.

Alzheimer responded to Erb's call and made it as far the south coast of France with the critically ill patient. But he could not cure him, and Geisenheimer died shortly thereafter in St. Raphael.

In the following period Alzheimer took tender care of his widow, Cecilie Simonette Nathalie Geisenheimer, née Wallerstein. She was not especially pretty, but as one of her granddaughters says of her, "Cecilie was a highly educated woman with great heartfelt kindness. Through her great journeys around the world she was open to all kinds of experience and she was wonderfully generous." Cecilie once said, certainly in reference to herself, "Beautiful hair and teeth are attributes of the ugly," but this was unquestionably an exaggeration because Cecilie was not ugly at all; she had a slender waist and was always elegantly dressed.

Alzheimer and Cecilie Geisenheimer became close, and one day the plucky woman took the initiative in asking him to marry her. In April 1894 the couple was married at the Frankfurt registry office. Franz Nissl, Alzheimer's loyal friend, was one of the witnesses, and businessman Alexander Strauss was the other. Through this marriage Alois Alzheimer became financially independent: Cecilie was wealthy and generous.

Rhine salmon and caviar were served after the civil wedding ceremony to a small circle of guests in the amply stocked house at 53 Liebiger Strasse (which is owned today by the pharmaceutical company Novartis). Cecilie's maid, Frieda Eiermann, who constantly accompanied her for, among other things, the care of her hair and wardrobe, later told Cecilie's daughters, "I know only this: It sounded Frankfurt-ish. Once I went with her to the train station, there she opened up her purse and took out a hundred-mark note and gave it to me."[36]

A hundred marks at the turn of the nineteenth century was a small fortune for a maid. Every day Cecilie had herself driven by a coach drawn by black horses into the inner city to go shopping.

To be married by the church as well as the state, Cecilie, of Jewish birth, converted to Christianity, which was problematic for her. Almost nine months passed until a church wedding could take place on February 14, 1895, in the chapel of the Frankfurt Franciscan nuns. It was high time because she could no longer conceal that the due date for their first child was imminent. For Alois and Cecilie it was important to receive the blessing of the Catholic Church before the birth.

Four weeks later, on March 10, 1895, Gertrud was born. Nissl became her godfather. Here again, no expense was spared. The honeymoon took the couple and their newborn to Italy. The newlyweds bought a Renaissance chest that they especially liked and sent it home; the family still owns it today.

Back in Frankfurt the Alzheimers entertained lavishly, as can be inferred from the notes of one of the granddaughters: "Hospitality was highly valued in the Alzheimer home; Cecilie knew how to make every visitor feel like a special guest. The apartment was exclusively furnished because in the course of her travels she visited a lot of museums, where, at that time, it was still possible to shop. She had impoverished science students tutored privately to make their studies easier. She employed eight servants, whom she treated very well."

In the same year Nissl moved to Heidelberg to do scientific work with Emil Kraepelin, director of the university psychiatric clinic. Despite the new, almost unlimited possibilities for his work, Nissl found the parting difficult. He and Alzheimer had become very close between 1889 and 1895:

I was always grateful to fate that it brought me together with a colleague who was so enthusiastic about science and that Sioli so eagerly supported our common scientific efforts. I acquainted Alzheimer with my technique and with slide preparations, and the experimental results convinced him that my views were correct, although at that time they were still not generally accepted at all. The goal of our efforts was always clear-cut: to understand the essential part of the pathological process of our mentally ill patients.[37]

In the Heidelberg clinic Nissl immediately monopolized the microphotographic laboratory that had been established at Kraepelin's initiative. From then on Nissl preferred microphotography to drawings because of its objectivity. He constantly feared the subjective because "one sees in a rather unpleasant and persistent way that which one believes oneself to have understood intellectually."[38]

The equipment was primitive and cumbersome by today's standards; the camera was large enough to accommodate a person, and the researcher had to work inside it. During his visits to Heidelberg Alzheimer spent many nights there, although because of his size he could work only in a crouching position. At the Heidelberg clinic every physician produced photographs and slide preparations himself. The only assistant was a disabled patient who also looked after the laboratory animals.

The short distance between Heidelberg and Frankfurt made possible numerous meetings of the two friends, during which Nissl reported at length on his work with the large equipment (although he had to leave his cigar outside when "microscoping" inside the camera) and tried to convince Alzheimer of the value of the new technique. Nissl later enthused,

> The mutual give and take of the old days in Frankfurt were renewed in these hours. . . . During one of his visits in Heidelberg I succeeded in convincing him—and Alzheimer was a first-class microscopic draftsman—of the usefulness of microphotography. It was Kraepelin, more than anyone, who must be credited with introducing the use of microphotography into the microtechniques of the central nervous system. We never just chattered at random. Alzheimer brought his slide preparations along, and I showed him mine.[39]

With Nissl's departure, the position of chief physician became vacant, and Alois Alzheimer applied for the job.[40] He wrote a letter, dated October 6, 1895, and directed it to the "highly commendable municipal authorities" of the city of Frankfurt am Main:

> The most obedient undersigned permits himself most respectfully to submit his application for the position of chief physician at the Mental Asylum at Frankfurt announced as open for application in the *Berliner Wochenschrift* of the first of the month.
>
> The undersigned permits himself, in his respectful request to be considered in the selection of a chief physician, specially to justify his application in that he is already in many ways familiar with the difficult and peculiar medical service in the local asylum, through what will soon be seven years of activity there, and his many years of experience will no doubt facilitate his doing justice to the duties of chief physician. Furthermore, because it has be-

come increasingly customary practice throughout Germany that doctors in mental asylums in the circle of a narrow group move into the higher vacated positions, it has become difficult, if not impossible, for a doctor employed at a city mental asylum to attain a higher position in his specialized calling elsewhere, even when he has made every effort to acquire the necessary knowledge and expertise to do so.

He included his medical license, a curriculum vitae, and a recommendation from Dr. Sioli. The first passages of the curriculum vitae are identical to those of his application papers from 1888, merely expanded by another paragraph:

In December 1888 he began as an intern in the local mental asylum, where he has worked without interruption until today. He used whatever time was left him after completion of his institutional duties in brain anatomic and clinical studies, the results of which he partly conveyed in lectures and partly published in psychiatric journals. The following articles have all been completed in the course of the last year and are in press:

—On a case of spinal progressive muscle atrophy with supervening disease of the bulbar nucleus (lecture in the Frankfurt Medical Association, *Archiv für Psychiatrie* [*Archive for Psychiatry*], Vol. 23)

—On the relationship between general paresis and syphilis (lecture to Frankfurt Medical Association)

—The arteriosclerotic atrophy of the brain (lecture at the Association of German Psychiatrists in Dresden, 1894)

—Juvenile paresis (lecture at the Conference of German Doctors and Scientists in Vienna, 1894)

—Colloidal degeneration of the brain (lecture at the Conference of German Psychiatrists in Hamburg, 1895)

—The early form of paresis

—Liepmann's pressure vision

—On a case of syphilitic meningomyelitis and meningoencephalitis.

Emil Sioli's recommendation stated that Alzheimer's "accomplishments in this job throughout this difficult time, which included a complete renovation of the asylum with a constantly overfilled occupancy and a renewal of the entire care personnel, have been absolutely exemplary and outstanding":

> Dr. Alzheimer has shown himself in every respect—in the training and supervision of a large staff as well as in the careful, humane treatment of his patients, for whom he goes to endless trouble, as well as in every aspect of medical knowledge and higher scientific effort—to be an exquisitely talented doctor imbued with the highest love for his profession and of a proven diligence in all his professional activities. He has acquired an extremely thorough psychiatric knowledge and a sure judgment in psychiatric-forensic matters and has so trained himself in the many relations that the special principles of acting in company with the patients and their relatives make necessary—a rather special spiritual kindness along with a proven firmness—as the Frankfurt Mental Asylum involves, that in the opinion of the undersigned director the asylum can only be congratulated if, after the departure of the current chief physician, it can employ Dr. Alzheimer in his place.

On October 21, 1895, Sioli forwarded the application documents to the Social Services Office. In an accompanying letter he spoke about "the demands placed by service in the local asylum . . . in dealing with patients of the most diverse classes and in public":

> Therefore there can be no doubt for the undersigned that under the remaining, otherwise equal applications, he deserves preference as one who has known the idiosyncrasies of the establishment for years, who has completely accustomed himself to them and has already served the asylum to its benefit and satisfaction for many years. I therefore make the request to the Social Services Office that from among the applicants for the chief physician position it propose the current intern of the local mental asylum, Dr. Alzheimer, to the municipal authorities for the appointment to the chief physician position.

On December 26, 1895, the city council responded with a resolution and thereby sealed the appointment procedure by declaring its agreement that the "position of chief physician of the mental asylum henceforth be occupied contractually at a mutual three-month notice with an annual salary of 3000 marks, the raising of which after each five years to 3500 marks and 4000 marks is taken into consideration, as well as a guarantee of housing provided by the institution, light and heating, which privileges are to be calculated upon retirement at 1000 marks, and apart from that so carried out that in this relation the forthcoming general regulations on contractual employment are applicable. The position named in paragraph 1 should be transferred to Dr. Alzheimer under the herewith specified conditions."

A caveat from Sioli about having a consulting practice delayed the completion of the contract; Sioli did "not want to hinder the chief physician from having some form of private practice—that will not be an issue given the full work demands in the asylum—but rather to ensure in urgent cases in which the director's deputy is desired for the sake of a mentally ill patient because the director is absent or unable to attend, the deputy makes this possible without delay."

However, this did not bother Alzheimer. Through his marriage to the wealthy widow Geisenheimer he had become so financially independent that later, when he moved with Kraepelin to Munich, he worked at the clinic free of charge. He already paid the costs for his publications and their numerous accompanying elaborate illustrations out of his own pocket.

Before Nissl's departure to Heidelberg the Alzheimers threw him a glittering farewell party. Alzheimer himself spoke rarely about money, preferring instead to hand it out generously.

Many documents from the time show just how bureaucratically things were run in Frankfurt. Papers from Social Services had to be approved by the municipal authorities. Consequently, Alois Alzheimer did not become chief physician of the Frankfurt Mental Asylum until July 21, 1896; the report of the Asylum for the Insane and Epileptic gives the details:

Multiple changes in the official personnel of the asylum have taken place since the appearance of the last full report. In October

1895 the chief physician, Dr. Franz Nissl, left us after six and a half years of work in the asylum to turn to a scientific career and to work toward his *Habilitation* in Heidelberg.

Dr. Nissl combined the most enthusiastic scientific efforts with complete and pure dedication to his calling, as well as strenuous work at the same, and proved himself a shining example for all of the younger doctors. We thank him here for his self-sacrificing work and express sincere good wishes for his future. His place was taken by Dr. A. Alzheimer, for many years the first intern. With the opening of the branch asylum in fall 1895 a new intern position was established, which was assigned to Mr. Friedrich Resch. Mr. Max Sander entered the position of first intern made vacant through Alzheimer's promotion.

The city of Frankfurt used the new district asylum as a nursing institution for impoverished patients. This reduced the number of patients at the Frankfurt Asylum for the Insane and Epileptic. Documents reveal that fifty patients were transferred there on October 28, 1896, and more patients in later years. Auguste D. was also supposed to be moved to the branch, but Alzheimer prevented it.

On July 23, 1896, Alzheimer's son, Hans, was born. Cecilie was so weakened by the birth that she had to leave Frankfurt to recover, but she arranged to be informed in precise detail about the baby's growth. Hans remembers what was often told him:

> Weight increases had to be telegraphed daily to mother: "Hans 5 gr," "Hans 10 gr," and so on. The post office official asked one day, "Excuse me, but is Hans a canary?" One of the eight servants was exclusively occupied with starching the baby's clothing for his afternoon outings in the pram.[41]

One of Hans Alzheimer's earliest childhood memories is the 1899 New Year's Eve party:

> The custom of greeting the new year with a lot of noise is found among all peoples. We had a large official residence on the Frankfurt *Affenstein* just next to the clinic, with a spacious terrace. On

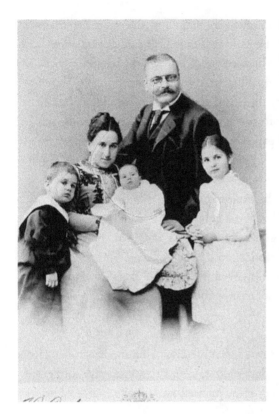

FIGURE 4.6 *Cecilie and Alois Alzheimer with their children, Hans, Maria, and Gertrud*

the terrace stood a small cannon; it was shining brass, as I had already established days earlier with Sioli's younger son.

That night I was brought to my parents on the terrace. The clinic personnel and friends were also assembled and an eager, playful mood reigned. Suddenly everyone put on fantastic masks, crouched on the ground, and then it was quiet as a mouse—then a flash—thundering, and with a cry everyone stood up and kissed: the year 1900 had begun.

Alzheimer could justifiably look back on his life with pride and satisfaction. He had big plans for the coming century. Although Sioli's clinic was not attached to a university, it was clear to Alzheimer that scientific work received strong support there. He later explained in his retrospective on the occasion of the twenty-fifth anniversary of Sioli's directorship of the Frankfurt Mental Asylum,

Alongside many institutions today that allow the desire for scientific research to flourish equally with medical care can be found a much larger number where research follows far behind day-to-day medical service and administrative activities. In reality, however, it is not clear why the better asylum doctor would not be one who, alongside his professional work, also strives to foster the scientific foundations of psychiatry. In any case, he will thereby receive much stimulation and joy from his profession.

There are many questions that cannot be explored in university clinics or that can be explored there only with far more difficulty than with the aid of the steady and abundant material of the larger asylums. Then gradually a deeper relationship between science and psychiatric practice could open up again, which we often miss today, one that would certainly benefit both sides and would make possible a faster solution to the tasks that we will face in the next twenty-five years.

Alois Alzheimer imagined his professional future in similar terms: combining clinical practice and science, as in Frankfurt, with further psychiatric research with the aid of the microscope, to take charge of his own mental asylum one day.

At this point, he could be well satisfied. In addition to his thesis he had published more than twenty articles in reputable journals and had given lectures at the annual specialty conferences that always received widespread recognition. He was highly esteemed at all the university clinics and large asylums, and his advice was often sought. He was happily married to Cecilie; they had two children, a daughter and a son; and another child was on the way, due in August 1900.

The year 1900 also was a good one for the Asylum for the Insane and Epileptic. Along with the director there were four salaried doctors active in the institution, so that there was one doctor for every eighty-five patients. Sioli and Alzheimer rigorously continued to remodel their "mental asylum" into a modern clinic. The isolation of patients became increasingly unnecessary because of the extensive use of duration baths; in addition to the cleansing baths and short medicinal baths, six tubs were available on both the men's and the women's sides, and they were used almost continuously. The 1899 report claims,

Through the use of duration baths we can keep a large number of the patients with melancholic, manic, catatonic, and paretic states of agitation in the bath during the day and in bed at night, in an individual room with an open door, without using narcotic means, whereas without the bath one could hardly avoid isolation or the use of narcotics.

Because coercive means are not necessary to keep patients in the bath, those responsible at the Frankfurt clinic see the use of prolonged baths as an extremely efficacious means of treating more serious motor states of agitation as well as in preventing and treating bedsores, the more rapid healing and cuticularization of larger wound surfaces, and fostering the healing of wounds subsequent to ulceration in paretic patients.

The doctors could counter the city administration's objection that operating costs could increase through the additional use of water by pointing to substantial savings on linen, which until then had been torn up by restless patients.

The number of "patients enjoying free movement" had also increased substantially, from 12 percent in the year 1897–98 to 34 percent of the asylum inmates in the year 1900. The open-door system was introduced in the calm and semicalm units, as well as the reception area and paretic wards; only the units for pensioners and the restless had closed doors. However, in the men's reception area it proved necessary to shut the doors again because the tremendous freedom was especially abused by alcoholics and patients with acute psychotic symptoms.

Paraldehyde and chloral were used as sedatives when necessary; bromine salts and often the Flechsig cure, a combined opium and bromine treatment, were prescribed for the epileptics; and for the melancholics opium or hyoscine often was used. Hyoscine, or scopolamine, is an opium alkaloid, generally injected beneath the surface of the skin and used primarily in cases of extreme agitation and flight of ideas. However, the doctors did recognize the dangers of habituation, and the annual report of the Asylum for the Insane and Epileptic remarks,

Ever-decreasing use has been made of hyoscine in recent years and then only in a combination with morphine, which appears substantially to reduce the unpleasant side effects of hyoscine. When we were compelled to use hyoscine in most cases it was associated with an extraordinary overcrowding in the institution. . . . Morphine also usually was used only temporarily in cases of extreme states of fear and peripherally caused pain.

Newly admitted patients generally were malnourished. They were helped, at first, by the plentiful and balanced nourishment given them in the asylum. Apart from the usual artificial nutrient preparations, used for more serious nutritional disorders, there was plenty of milk, butter, and eggs.

Thus, for example, on March 31, 1901, there were extra prescriptions of 330 portions of milk at half a liter each, 83 portions of cacao, 22 portions of bouillon, 353 eggs, 13 open sandwiches, 23 rusks, 4 portions of pudding, 33 portions of butter, 13 portions of soup, 83 portions of beer, 39 portions of wine, and 84 small bottles of soda water.

In the unit predominantly for treating drinkers, there were no alcoholic beverages. The epileptics also received neither wine nor beer. However, the institution was not subject to complete abstinence because the doctors saw no harm in light beer and wine consumed in moderation:

> We had to regard the withdrawal of a popular and safe semi-luxury food as a kind of coercive measure, the implementation of which had reason only in medically imperative cases. For many melancholics and many forms of senile sleeplessness alcohol in the form of beer proved to be a valuable soporific. Among some patients the Russian Kvas enjoyed great popularity; because of its very low alcohol content, low cost, refreshing effect, and ease of production it deserves general distribution.

Of course, interpersonal relationships were also fostered; family bonds were promoted through relatives' visits: "They have increased from 9000 to 10,000 in 1897–98 to now more than 12,000" according to the annual report of 1900.

Sioli and Alzheimer could be proud of what they had achieved since 1888 through to the end of the nineteenth century.

## 1901: A Fateful Year

For Alzheimer, 1901 was a fateful year. In his professional environment things were continuing to look up. Thanks in part to his great commitment, the Asylum for the Insane and Epileptic was expanded with the addition of a branch institution. The year 1901 also saw his first encounter with Auguste D. However, before all this the greatest catastrophe of his entire life occurred: the death of his beloved wife, Cecilie.

Her illness began in early 1901 with a mild throat inflammation; later symptoms included pain in the limbs and signs of kidney disease. Cecilie could no longer run the household, and Alzheimer had to ask his sister, Elisabeth, for help. Nevertheless, Cecilie set firm rules for their cohabitation. In January 1901, a month before her death, she wrote,

> Your brother has instructed me to reply to your letter to him; he is very busy at the moment. You ask whether you can be received into our household. We have discussed it, and we welcome you sincerely. But Alzheimer asks you in the strongest terms to consider that you have to keep your religious ideas to yourself, as we do ours, so that the peace of the family is not disturbed.
>
> Maria is already eating off a spoon in the cutest of ways, Gertrud and Hans have had bad colds; it will be good when everything calms down again. We want to go to the seaside in the summer, for the children.

That did not happen. Although leading experts from Frankfurt were consulted, they could not prevent Cecilie's early death, the cause of which remains unknown.

Elisabeth promised the dying Cecilie to care for the children and take over the household. Despite her severe manner, she eventually became the warmly beloved "Maja" to the children; she also brought up their children and helped care for the fourth generation by doing a lot of knitting. She died at age 96.

Cecilie was solemnly laid to rest in the main cemetery in Frankfurt on February 28, 1901. The gravestone, made specially for them by Berlin sculptor Fritz Klimsch, today also covers the grave of Alois Alzheimer.

The same sculptor was commissioned in 1910 to make a memorial for the famous Rudolf Virchow. It resembles the gravestone for Cecilie Alzheimer: Both monuments show double figures that allegorically represent the struggle of life with death.

The grave lies on the wall with the Jewish cemetery so that Cecilie lies near her family, the Wallersteins, who were buried directly on the other side.

The eldest daughter of the Alzheimers, Gertrud, later reminisced happily about her mother, who often let her children run free: "In the attic there was a mysterious, large suitcase from overseas that we children rummaged through with great curiosity. A wonderful scent, perhaps musk, gushed from it, and splendid clothes and robes were kept in there. When as a young girl now and then I played theater and was allowed to put on this wonderful dress with blue-black shimmering sequins, as well as an ostrich-feather fan and lace umbrella, then, although I was thin, I would have to hold my breath so that all of the hooks closed."

Alzheimer's son, Hans, also remembers his mother well: "I often sat closely snuggled up to her in a black coach drawn by black horses; I was so happy." He also has vague memories from the time after his mother's death: "My bed stood in my father's room. If I awoke during the night, I saw father sitting at the writing desk, lit by the lamp. 'What did you dream, Hänser?' he asked me in a warm, soothing voice. And with that all childhood fears vanished and I felt safe."

With Cecilie's death life in the house changed fundamentally; the "wonderful generosity" that had prevailed until then was abruptly over. One of the granddaughters wrote, "Baja immediately took her task to hand: seven servants were fired and the upbringing of the children became strictly Catholic. For example, when you lied, your mouth had to be washed out with soap, or when a child lashed out at the parents, he [was told that he] deserved to have the hand chopped off."

Another granddaughter reported, "The lifestyle became bourgeois" and a third, who characterized Elisabeth's way as "petit-bourgeois and overly pious," remarked, "Alois wanted to know that his children were well taken care of and let Elisabeth prevail to the greatest possible extent. After such a happy marriage with Cecilie he did not want to marry again, so he plunged himself into his work."

Alzheimer was inexhaustibly active at the asylum, where he also carried out examinations outside the normal hours of his rounds. He carefully wrote up his case histories, attended to stacks of patient files, took on the time-consuming tasks of a court-appointed expert, and continued his beloved histologic studies with even greater passion. On the outside he did not let anyone notice his mourning; on the contrary, he met the many demands of his work with a kind composure.

A great deal of his energy was absorbed by work for the new branch asylum. Sioli had already worked on the idea of establishing a rural "Colony for the Insane" away from the city in 1881, and in 1901, together with his chief physician, he realized the idea in Köppern, near Frankfurt.

On February 23, 1901, just a few days before Cecilie's death, the municipal authorities of the city of Frankfurt, supported by the report of the Social Welfare Office, gave the Asylum for the Insane and Epileptic approval to acquire the iron and steel mill at Köppern in Taunus and the property needed to realign the boundaries and expand the mental asylum, at a total cost of 151,000 marks. It was fortunate for the asylum that on January 1, 1901, factory owner Ludo Mayer and his wife, Luise, née Henle, had made available 5000 marks for the "establishment of a free-bed foundation for curable needy patients."

The new branch asylum was not meant to be further from the main asylum than would allow medical supervision from Frankfurt and would permit patients to be visited by their relatives without great expenditure of time and money. The asylum in Köppern at first was occupied only by Frankfurt patients, and for this reason the tie to the main asylum was important. But the mentally ill patients without means, for whom no asylum was available at all, were especially close to Sioli's heart:

There is the concern about the great number of patients who, on one hand, do not belong in the mental asylums but, on the other hand, are also not in the right place in the general hospitals because they cannot receive the correct and appropriate treatment there. Whereas a large number of psychiatric and cold-water institutions are available to the nervous patients who belong to the well-off and wealthy circles of the population, there is no appropriate place of refuge for the many ill who are without means or rely on public health where they can find longer-term treatment and healing from their often serious complaints.[42]

In a memorandum Sioli enthused,

The location of the purchased land is one of the most beautiful around Frankfurt, admittedly 27 kilometers outside of the city, but on the southeast slope of the Taunus mountains, on the edge of the romantically situated Köppern Valley, twenty minutes above the village of Köppern, with the Erlen brook on both sides. This stream, which originates from the north side of the Feldberg more than 500 meters above sea level, at first takes a long course over the Taunus plateau through meadows abounding in water, then enters the Köppern valley at 330 meters above sea level. This extends as a gorge-like cleft of steep slopes of two mountain chains, bordered in part by stony falls, from west to east from the mill up to the steel mill.[43]

The "Colony for the Insane" project proved so convincing that Alzheimer was invited to give a lecture that led, on October 1, 1902, to the opening of a detoxification center on the castle hill at Biber by the Regional Association Against the Abuse of Alcoholic Drinks of Kassel–Frankfurt–Wiesenbaden–Darmstadt.

The catering for our wards happens almost exclusively with the means of the estate. Good uncontaminated whole milk from cows that are kept in the open air, fresh butter, fresh eggs, home-cultivated vegetables. Honey from bees from our own apiary, meat from pigs, calves, and sheep we have slaughtered ourselves—we offer all of this so that the patient's usually weakened body becomes strong again.

Good reading and communal entertainment evenings should further harmoniously influence the convalescence of the patients. Depending on profession and strength, patients are given activities in the fields, pastures or farming, and are thus reaccustomed to regular work, which many have not practiced for a long time.[44]

The costs of care of 130 to 180 marks were payable quarterly. The wards had to submit to a strict house order that did not permit them to leave the institution for the first three months. During subsequent excursions they were not permitted to visit pubs or drink alcohol; indeed, even letters, packages, newspapers, and books were subject to the censorship and control of the house father. In case of violations, Alzheimer emphasized, the house father had the right to expel the ward from the institution immediately.

## 5. To Munich via Heidelberg

A widower at thirty-seven, Alois had to think about his future. There was nothing to keep him in Frankfurt anymore. At first Alzheimer did not think about an academic career as much as work in a clinical institution, as director of which he could have combined theoretical research with practice.

His application for the directorship of a regional institution in 1902 was rejected, and in retrospect one could describe this rejection as fortunate. Emil Kraepelin heard about it, and in his memoirs Kraepelin wrote, "It was very lucky for him that he did not succeed with his application."[1] Alzheimer was very disappointed about the failure of his plan to become director of an asylum, but things ended well: Kraepelin convinced Alzheimer to come and work with him in Heidelberg.

Alzheimer's best friend and colleague, Franz Nissl, had finished his *Habilitation* there and become an unsalaried professor in 1901. He advised Alzheimer, even urged him in a telephone conversation, to move to Heidelberg. To convince Alzheimer, Nissl might have raised as a reason something that appears in his notebooks: "The psychiatry that I knew until now and myself conducted 'scientifically' was not science at all. Only here in Heidelberg did the light go on for me, letting me see a truly scientific clinical psychiatry. And for that I thank Kraepelin."[2]

Alzheimer resigned his service in Frankfurt. They were reluctant to let him go, as is made clear by Sioli's report of the Asylum for the Insane and Epileptic at Frankfurt from April 1, 1898, to March 31, 1903:

> To our great regret Dr. Alzheimer, for many years the chief physician of the institution, left his position with us on March 1 of this year to devote himself to scientific studies in Heidelberg. He started work here at the local asylum as an intern on December 1, 1888, and has been active as chief physician since November 1, 1895.

Inexhaustible in his work for the well-being of the patients and full of keen interest in the development of the asylum, for many years he devoted the best of his labors here to the care of the insane and prepared and made possible the extraordinary upturn that this care has taken through his inexhaustible sense of responsibility and his personal care for every individual patient. . . .

The patients, the authorities, the younger doctors who will have to forgo his stimulating guidance, the courts that regard his careful expert testimony so highly, all regret his departure. Numerous scientific works, which he published while based here, demonstrate his continuous scientific efforts. The increased external burden of work, which made scientific research increasingly difficult, contributed to Dr. Alzheimer's decision to leave. We retain a sincere feeling of gratitude for his many years of cooperation and wish him the best success in the scientific field.

Alzheimer's departure from Sioli was not easy for either man; they held each other in great professional esteem and always understood each other well throughout Alzheimer's fifteen years in Frankfurt. Sioli promised to keep Alzheimer up to date on the most interesting cases, especially the case of Auguste D.

The small laboratory in Heidelberg, which Alzheimer knew well from many visits to Nissl, attracted him above all because of the international research community assembled there. It was made up of the leading figures in psychiatry and included Ugo Cerletti, who later became *Ordinarius* (full professor) of psychiatry in Rome, C. B. Farrar from the United States, M. C. Campbell from England, A. Debaux from France, H. Evensen from Norway, and G. Biondi from Switzerland.

Thus Alzheimer's wish for a laboratory with international contacts and exchanges of opinion was fulfilled. However, the conditions in the Heidelberg clinic were less gratifying; Kraepelin describes them as follows:

Patient transfers were held up because the health care institutions were filled to capacity; we could no longer empty the clinic promptly but were nevertheless compelled to take care of ever more patients, which naturally led to the grossest inadequacies.

Not only were all the beds constantly occupied, but it was also increasingly necessary to let patients sleep on mattresses on the floor. Because we could most easily get rid of quiet patients, the especially restless ones piled up to such an intolerable degree that there could be little proper care; instead, patients, nursing staff, and doctors all suffered equally from the impossibility of creating the urgently needed calm and order.

It happened that with the number of patients for whose daily board we were compensated with only 1.50 marks, the economic condition of the clinic progressively declined. In the first years it had been possible for me to achieve large annual surpluses through an appropriate admixture of better-paying patients. This was useful for the improvement of our facilities and particularly for our scientific efforts. However, the developments I have described led inexorably to growing deficits, which made attaining special approvals increasingly difficult.[3]

The conditions at Kraepelin's clinic became increasingly unproductive. The scientific environment was gratifyingly rigorous under the influence of his excellent colleagues, but the "intolerable overcrowding increased further, so that it was no longer possible even to think about well-ordered care for the patients."

It was at this troubled time that the report of the death of Anton Bumm arrived. Bumm had assumed the directorship of the Psychiatric Clinic and the District Mental Asylum in Munich in 1896. Although in 1901 Bumm had resigned the leadership of the asylum, he had retained the professorship and dedicated himself to the planned new construction of the university psychiatric clinic, the completion of which he did not live to see.

Kraepelin was deeply upset by Bumm's death, but as a former student of Gudden he also hoped to be called to Munich. "I therefore had to fear that I could face the decision as to whether I wanted, despite my decided disinclination, to come to terms with the ills I struggled against or whether I would have to give up my professorship in favor of the Munich position."[4]

In June 1903, Kraepelin was offered the appointment. He definitely wanted to take Alzheimer with him to Munich. He also convinced Robert

FIGURE 5.1  *Emil Kraepelin*

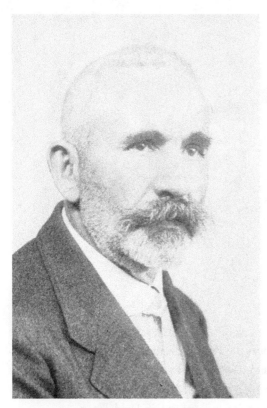

Gaupp to join them; Gaupp had written his *Habilitation* on dipsomania under Kraepelin. Thus, after a brief stay in Heidelberg that reunited him with
his old friend Nissl, Alzheimer followed Kraepelin to Munich at the beginning of October 1903. Gaupp followed a year later.

Before Alzheimer left Heidelberg, he sent his curriculum vitae and his
bibliography, both handwritten, to Munich. The bibliography contained
seventeen publications; the first part of the curriculum vitae was unchanged
from the earlier versions but concluded,

> In order to be able to devote himself more to scientific studies,
> in March 1903 he left the position of chief physician at the Mu-
> nicipal Mental Asylum in Frankfurt, after *Hofrat* Prof. Kraepelin
> had promised him a position as a scientific assistant at his clinic
> in Heidelberg. Like Prof. Kraepelin, he moved in October of
> this year to Munich.[5]

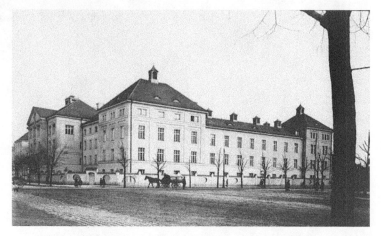

FIGURE 5.2 *The Royal Psychiatric Clinic in Munich*

## New Tasks

The year 1903 was a troubled one for Alzheimer, yet it was also a crucial one for his future. First of all, it was the year he decided to accept Kraepelin's offer and go to Heidelberg, and it was the year he gained a completely new perspective in Munich. However, this meant that he could no longer hand in his *Habilitation* thesis, an extensive manuscript, in Heidelberg.

Through constant travels between Frankfurt and Heidelberg and many fact-finding trips to Munich Alzheimer could not produce his accustomed number of publications or attend as many meetings as he used to.

Alzheimer had enough time on the train ride from Heidelberg to Munich to inform himself about the Royal Psychiatric Clinic of the Ludwig-Maximilian University at Munich. He already knew the biography of his new boss: Emil Kraepelin was six years older than he and came from Neustrelitz in Mecklenburg. Kraepelin had also studied medicine in Würzburg and passed the *Physikum* and the state exams there. But whereas Alzheimer had remained in the same place—Frankfurt—for fifteen years, Kraepelin had expanded his horizons at various training sites: the District Mental Asylum in Munich with von Gudden, the Leipzig Psychiatric Clinic with Paul Flechsig, and the Psychiatric and Outpatient Clinic in Heidelberg with Wilhelm Erb.

At the suggestion of Wilhelm Wundt, by 1883 Kraepelin had already written his *Compendium of Psychiatry*, and soon his psychiatry textbooks were known worldwide. In 1884 he started his clinical career with von Gudden at the District Mental Asylum in Munich, then went to Dresden as directing doctor of the mental unit of the general hospital and later became a professor of psychiatry in Dorpat (now called Tartu, in Estonia) and then went to Heidelberg.

This career impressed Alzheimer, and he looked forward to working with Kraepelin, especially because he also saw the chance to smooth his own path to a university professorship through collaboration with this outstanding figure.

The history of the Munich clinic began early: The Holy Spirit Hospital was founded in 1200; 600 years later, troubling conditions still prevailed. Until 1803 the mentally ill were put in the *Keiche*, as the fifth unit of the hospital was called. This was a separate building and was meant to hold about thirty patients, but in 1803 it housed sixty-four. In 1781 there were only twenty-four "complete and half idiots" present, of whom two died and three recuperated. All of the horrors of medieval mental asylums prevailed; at the beginning of the nineteenth century, chains could still be seen on the walls.

The tragic conditions were vividly described in *A History of Munich Hospitals and Clinics*, a book published in 1913:

> Instead of clean canvas, instead of light bedding, I saw many in terrible rags and beds shoved together into a pile. The healthiest person would get sick here in a few weeks, and this is where the sick are supposed to be cured? And who could even guess that in two large and connected cellar-like, low-ceilinged caves that lie below street level can be found forty-three men in one and eighty-six women in another?[6]

In 1601 Prince Maximilian I had the Herzogs Hospital built on what is today Herzog-Spital Strasse; it contained several rooms for psychotic patients who could not be put in the Holy Spirit Hospital.[7]

The "court hospital," a third institution, was originally intended for treating court officials with acute infectious diseases; it was used from 1803 on as a psychiatric clinic and was popularly known, after the suburb where it was located, as the "Giesing Madhouse."

Until 1837, in accordance with a law decreed by King Ludwig I that allocated responsibility for psychiatric care to the districts, the Giesing court hospital was converted into a psychiatric clinic, the Upper Bavarian District Mental Asylum. The first director of this clinic, from 1864 to 1872, was Karl August von Solbrig, who also occupied the first chair of psychiatry at the Ludwig-Maximilian University in Munich.

Alzheimer very much liked the ground plan of the District Mental Asylum; it reminded him of Hoffmann's clinic on the *Affenstein*. The female patients were housed on the left wing, the men on the right. Certainly Heinrich Hoffmann was already well acquainted with the Upper Bavarian District Mental Asylum when during a vacation he made an extensive series of visits to mental asylums in Germany and Austria.

Solbrig's successor was Bernhard von Gudden, director of the Upper Bavarian District Mental Asylum from 1872 to 1886. In an unpublished curriculum vitae Nissl reported on the von Gudden clinic: "The exemplary organization and the working of the District Mental Asylum made a powerful impression on me. . . . One learned from von Gudden how to deal with the mentally ill. For me the deep seriousness with which he conceived of his task as a psychiatrist, the great respect shown to the humanity of mental patients, and the purposeful direction of a big institution, through which a fresh and happy spirit blew, is unforgettable. For us doctors von Gudden was incontestably the ideal example that we all sought to imitate." Yet Nissl adds, "However, one could not learn clinical psychiatry in the scientific sense from von Gudden."[8]

Alongside Nissl, Siegbert J. M. Ganser also worked in von Gudden's anatomic laboratory; Ganser's syndrome, a feigned imbecility, was named after him. Patients with Ganser's syndrome display a behavior that emerges as a reaction to the intolerable situation of their own helplessness; incorrect responses and apparent ignorance give it the appearance of a mental disorder. And Emil Kraepelin also worked in von Gudden's laboratory from 1884 to 1885.

Von Gudden was followed in 1886 by his son-in-law Hubert von Grashey, whom Alzheimer knew from his time in Würzburg, when von Grashey was director of the psychiatric unit of the Julius Hospital and *Ordinarius* of psychiatry. From von Grashey also comes an obituary of his father-in-law that clearly depicts the events and the unwitnessed, tragic end of King Ludwig II of Bavaria and his personal physician.

From 1899 to 1903 von Grashey's successor, Anton Bumm, planned and set up the new construction of the Psychiatric Clinic on Nussbaumstrasse; he died on April 13, 1903, after a gall bladder operation. He was succeeded by Kraepelin, who had requested during negotiations for his appointment the right to control the final execution of the building, although at issue were primarily the details of the interior furnishings. The ground plan and floor plan had already been largely established by his predecessor, Bumm.

Alzheimer also thought himself capable of contributing to the completion of the clinic; after all, in Frankfurt there had been continual renovation and expansion. Littmann, the architect, describes it as follows:

> In the form of a giant horseshoe . . . the institutional building extends from the corner of Goethestrasse and Nussbaumstrasse, from the municipal hospital left of the Isar River toward the northwest, adjoining and surrounded by numerous other institutions of the medical faculty of the university.
>
> The main building with a ground and three upper floors is 30 meters long on Nussbaumstrasse and contains in the middle a main entrance, which is distinguished by a covered access route in imitation shell limestone.
>
> Here the hedge wall, the oval and round archlike barred openings of which permit a view into the sprawling front gardens, arches back to the house. Three wings adjoin it: an east wing, 37 meters long, on the border with the hospital, with a top floor, a west wing on Goethestrasse, 45 meters long, with three top floors, and one in the middle.[9]

Alzheimer's anatomy laboratory was on the fourth floor of the clinic; he had already conceptualized the layout. There was a lot to do before the ceremonial opening the following year.

Until his family arrived Alzheimer took temporary lodgings in a hotel; on October 2, 1903, he registered himself as a resident and soon afterward found himself an apartment on the third floor of an 1870s, *Gründerzeit*-style house on Rükertstrasse, so that he lived just a hundred steps away from the clinic.

Because he was within hearing range of the clinic, he witnessed disturbances caused by a number of patients. Of course, Alzheimer was not the only one. A first-rate concert singer lodged a complaint with the state ministry: "For some time a number of raving mad mental patients have been housed in the psychiatric clinic; for about the past fourteen days they have made such an infernal noise every night from around half past ten in the evening until about five in the morning that not only are the occupants of the houses opposite the clinic robbed of their nightly rest, but larger crowds have also repeatedly formed in front of the psychiatric clinics."[10]

The Alzheimer's apartment was also not far from the *Theresienwiese*, the meadow where since 1815 the *Wies'n*, the Munich *Oktoberfest*, has taken place.

Alzheimer's family—the three children and his sister Elisabeth (Maja)—soon followed. Maja presided over the house and took care of the children. Whether she ever got around to taking the examination to become a handicraft teacher, as she had once intended, remains unknown. Meanwhile, she got used to family life, although she could never really cope with Alois's upper-class lifestyle.

On the other hand, she was completely fearless, as is shown by her leisure activity, rather uncommon at the time: She was one of the first female Zeppelin pilots. The first Zeppelin journey, of July 1, 1909, is described in a contemporary report: "This almost twelve-hour journey departed in the morning from Friedrichshafen, at first in a westerly direction over Stein am Rhein and Schaffhausen, turned in a large arc toward the southwest, from where the airship traveled over Zug in the direction of the Vierwaldstät Lake and reached a height of 750 meters." The trip was also historically unique because "for the first time two crowned heads, the king and queen of Württemberg, participated in this victory flight through the air."[11]

It did Alzheimer good to have to find his way around in a new place, and the many new tasks that took all of his strength helped him get over the loss of Cecilie.

The design of the Munich clinic was unfinished at the time of Bumm's death, so Kraepelin visited several of the newer clinics in Germany to get some new ideas.

He visited the Giesing clinic first, then traveled to Kiel, where he found a clinic that he especially liked, except for the wards for the restless patients. Finally he went to Halle to visit Eduard Hitzig's clinic. Hitzig, a friend of writer Gottfried Keller, had become director of the Burghölzli psychiatric hospital in Zürich in 1875 and was professor of psychiatry in

Halle-Nietleben from 1879 on; in 1891 he put into operation an exemplary new clinic in Giessen and was known as an excellent organizer.

Kraepelin and Alzheimer's important collaboration in the arrangement of the rooms and furnishings at the Munich clinic is verified by Kraepelin's memoirs: "Thus I was compelled, in months of strenuous work, during which I was supported by Alzheimer in the most conscientious and tireless manner, to pick every single requisite object according to kind, size, number, composition, and price myself."[12]

Later in his memoirs, he added this astounding passage: "Alzheimer entered the service of the clinic without pay because I did not have a position for him and because he wanted to be in charge of how he spent his time. To establish his affiliation with the clinic, I created the class of scientific assistant; it was supposed to include researchers who took advantage of the clinic's aid without remuneration. Apart from Alzheimer, Rüdin and Plaut, and later Isserling, worked under such an arrangement with the clinic.

Without the selfless help of these gentlemen it would have been completely impossible to put the scientific life of the clinic back on its feet. In this way, we succeeded in obtaining particularly outstanding specialists for a series of complementary sciences and thereby achieved a division of labor that signified a substantial development of research in the most diverse directions.

What is unthinkable today clearly was not unusual at the beginning of the twentieth century: scientific work without pay at a university institute. As a financially independent widower, Alzheimer could afford to work without compensation.

The second scientific assistant, Swiss-born Ernst Rüdin, became full professor of psychiatry in Munich in 1933 and a member of the specialist advisory council for population and racial policy in the Third Reich's Interior Ministry; he can be considered a pioneer of German "Hereditary and Racial Care."

The third in the group, Felix Plaut, in 1907 discovered the syphilitic origin of general paresis and in 1915 became leader of the serologic laboratory. His chief work, "Wassermann's Serodiagnosis with Regard to Syphilis and Its Application to Psychiatry," appeared in Jena in 1908.

The fourth, Max Isserlin, in 1926 wrote an important textbook on psychotherapy.

On November 7, 1904, almost exactly a year after Kraepelin and Alzheimer had begun their work in Munich, the clinic was ceremonially opened in the presence of the Minister for Education and the Arts and numerous guests.

Kraepelin gave the main speech, in which he offered an overview of almost half a century of clinical instruction in Munich and the many plans that had been developed for the construction of this clinic, which fortunately had not been carried out: "They would have stood in the way of the current, only proper solution." After the ceremonial opening the guests went on a tour of the completed rooms.

The Munich *Neuesten Nachrichten* of November 7 reported,

Today, Monday morning 11 o'clock, the new psychiatric clinic was officially declared open.

The participants at the opening celebrations assembled in the large lecture hall, where a colossal bust of the Prince Regent had been erected beneath richly adorned decorative plants. . . . The director of the institution, *Hofrat* Dr. Kraepelin, gave an account of the prehistory of the clinic in a one-hour lecture. Since 1863 the establishment of the clinic had repeatedly been contemplated and proposed, until in 1902 both chambers had approved the means for construction. The speaker movingly commemorated his predecessor, Dr. Anton Bumm, who saw the establishment of the clinic as his life's work, the completion of which he did not live to see. The facilities and layout of the clinic the speaker described as Bumm's work; he said that he himself had contributed only individual additions such as the duration baths.

Dr. Kraepelin then described in detail the institution's equipment and the treatment of patients according to modern psychiatric methods. At the end of his speech the speaker thanked the Minister of Education and the Arts, both chambers of the Medical Faculty of the City of Munich, and everyone who had helped in the work. At this point the tour through the rooms of the institution commenced. The approximately 300 people present undertook the inspection in seven groups with medical tour guides.

The institution is, as already briefly described elsewhere, equipped with all the needs of modern psychiatry and offers much of interest with regard to teaching materials as well as hygienic and therapeutic equipment. The modern treatment of the insane has completely departed from the isolation system, and the new clinic contains no actual isolation rooms. Empirical experience has presented a different approach: Quite serious cases, which one previously isolated, are treated in duration baths. The patients lie continuously for days, weeks, even months, according to the condition of the case, in warm baths, where, experience shows, they feel very comfortable and also behave calmly, almost without exception.

Intelligently conceived equipment in the bathtubs ensures that the patient has all the comforts. The greatest care is devoted to the furnishing of the baths in the new institution, corresponding to their outstanding importance in the modern treatment of the insane. The remaining rooms appointed for the stay of the patients, the bedrooms and the living rooms, also show taste. It is interesting to see how all precautionary measures have been taken to protect the patients from suicide and how the wretchedness of their condition is meant to be kept away from consciousness as much as possible.

The institution is set up in both of these directions down to the finest detail, one might even say with finesse. Everything reveals that a fine observer of the life of the sick mind is at work here. Patients are not locked up unless it is absolutely necessary, nor are the windows locked; patients have cozy, sensitively and artistically furnished day rooms in which they can enjoy complete freedom of movement, activity, and entertainment—everything, in short, that could allow the patient to forget the feeling of having to stay in the asylum compulsorily.

The arrangements for teaching are still in the early stages, but they should be complete within a few months. These are outfitted mostly according to the wishes of the psychiatric clinic's director, Privy Councillor Dr. Kraepelin. The room for microphotography aroused particular interest among the visitors.

This room is so arranged that the operator finds himself enclosed in the apparatus because the photographic plates are illuminated in the same room in which the operator acts. It would lead us too far afield to go into all the details of the equipment for microscopy, microphotography, anatomic slide preparations, and physiological examination.

Visitors to the clinic were also permitted to glance through the living spaces of the doctors, nine of whom work at the institution, as well as the living rooms of the Sisters of Charity, and the working quarters, which are entrusted to the care of the Charitable Sisters, who have also taken over the nursing in the psychiatric clinic. Everything is set up in an immensely practical and comfortable way and lets one forget completely the serious purpose the building serves.

In contrast, evidence of the frankly barbaric treatment of the insane of earlier times has a repulsive effect. Dr. Kraepelin presented his visitors in the institution with "means of treatment" of the insane, including various forms of straitjacket: "indestructible suits" that were made of the coarsest material—mostly burlap—with strong leather set on the neck and arm openings and were equipped with trick locks to make removal of the garment impossible.

This contrast splendidly illustrated Dr. Kraepelin's highly informative lecture on the modern hydrotherapeutic treatment of the insane, and the visitor left with the sense of being introduced to the secrets of the most serious of all professions by a man who is not only an outstanding expert but also a true philanthropist.[13]

Everyday life began immediately after the opening. A very active operation with almost 2000 admissions in the year was reported, and there were four salaried assistant doctors as well as a military doctor ordered by the war ministry to serve at the psychiatric clinic.

Volunteer doctors also were active there; three lived in house and two outside. A chief physician stood at Kraepelin's side as his deputy: initially Dr. Gaupp and later Dr. von Gudden, the son of one of his predecessors, who originally ran the outpatient clinic.

The outpatient clinic was on the second floor and was equipped with all the apparatuses needed for modern diagnostics and therapy for psychological illnesses, including a darkroom, an ophthalmoscope, and a complete box of glasses with Snell tables, on which were printed letters of distinct sizes for vision testing. For hearing examinations there was a complete set of tuning forks and an otoscope. A laboratory table with the necessary reagents for urine analysis and objects for testing the sense of touch were also available.

For therapeutic purposes there were electric vibration apparatuses and an electrostatic inducer. The annual report of the Royal Psychiatric Clinic in Munich also described both bathrooms, which contained "on the one side a full bath and the most effective showers, on the other side an electric full bath, the so-called Fayence bathtub, and a four-cell bath."

Kraepelin wrote of his co-workers, "Apart from Gaupp and Alzheimer, who took over the establishment and management of the incredibly well-equipped anatomic work rooms, I had only brought one doctor to Munich with me from Heidelberg, Dr. Nitsche, of whom I hoped above all that he should organize the peaceable and focused collaboration of the other doctors, who came from the most diverse fields."

From the records it also becomes clear how difficult the first year in Munich was:

> As a consequence of various unfavorable influences and also especially because of the large number of younger doctors, it became tremendously difficult for me to introduce into the workplace the spirit of enthusiasm for labor and science to which I aspired. Even the loyal help of my colleagues Gaupp and Alzheimer could not overcome these obstacles for a long time.
>
> The close personal relationships that had bound us together in our common work on the small scale of the Heidelberg clinic could not, despite all of my efforts in this direction, be reproduced. This lack of internal connection made my job all the more difficult.[14]

This quote from Kraepelin's memoirs reveals that a personal distance had opened up between Kraepelin and Alzheimer. Alzheimer increasingly realized this; he missed the warm interaction with Sioli that he had become accustomed to in Frankfurt and, above all, the friendship with Nissl.

## Venia Legendi

On November 16, 1903, after a month in Munich, living in Rükertstrasse and having already registered himself with the police, Alzheimer handed in

FIGURE 5.3 *Title page
of Alzheimer's Habilitation
thesis, "Differential Diagnosis
of General Paresis," 1904*

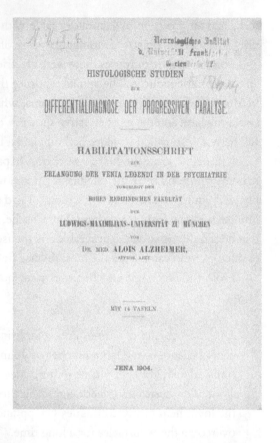

his *Habilitation* thesis to the Higher Medical Faculty of the Ludwig-Maximilian University in Munich and applied for the *venia legendi*, or permission to teach in the field of psychiatry.[15] The title of his work was "Histological Studies of General Paresis."[16]

He included his credentials along with the *Habilitation* thesis: the doctoral diploma and thesis, his medical license, a curriculum vitae, and a bibliography of his publications.

The early submission date shows that Alzheimer had arrived in Munich with the completed and printed thesis. In Frankfurt and Heidelberg, working tirelessly at night, he had reviewed and evaluated his results and recorded them in a 299-page text. Nissl had already said in Heidelberg that "the *Habilitation* represents the ripe fruit of work in the Frankfurt asylum." Still impressive today are the eleven elaborate illustrations that Alzheimer drew and colored himself, as well as the numerous photographs.

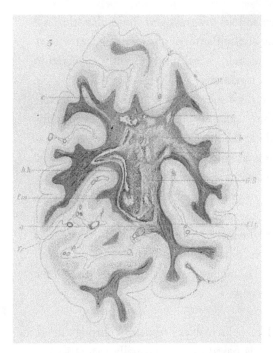

FIGURE 5.4 *Frontal section through the occipital lobe of a patient with arteriosclerotic dementia, drawn by Alzheimer (from the Habilitation thesis)*

The next day the office of the dean turned to *Hofrat* Dr. Emil Kraepelin, asking that he assume the responsibility of evaluating the *Habilitation* thesis and that senior medical counsel Prof. Dr. Otto von Bollinger co-evaluate the *Habilitation*. Why a delay arose is not known with any certainty.

Initially Alzheimer asked Kraepelin to send the documents back to the dean's office; obviously he wanted to postpone the matter. Perhaps the duties of his new position were so demanding that he did not have time to prepare his test lecture. In May 1904 Kraepelin requested that the office of the dean return the documents to begin the *Habilitation* procedure, and on June 16, 1904, he received the second evaluation from Bollinger. Kraepelin had only words of praise:

> The work at issue here is without doubt an extraordinary achievement. A frankly astonishing amount of the most strenuous individual labor is contained in these simply presented depictions of the most difficult aspect of the pathology of the cerebral cortex; the illustrations are exemplary in their clarity and completeness. The careful and comprehensive labeling of the individual anatomic

symptoms signifies tremendous progress and shows that, through the methodical, untiring accumulation of observations, knowledge can also be gained in this field, which until recently appeared to confound every probing treatment.

Above all, however, the writer has demonstrated the principle that pathological anatomy can also be an important, even indispensable aid in researching the theory of mental disorders. His attempt to place diverse anatomic images beside the finer clinical differences of individual disease processes distinguished by him, practically for the first time, makes it possible for psychiatry to appear to be equal to the other fields of medicine in its mode of research and its results. Alzheimer's monograph therefore will form basis for all similar efforts for a long time. It shows that its author is a mature researcher who unquestionably is prepared to join the teaching body of a university.

Bollinger agreed with Kraepelin in every respect: "Through the results of the work at hand, which is based on an unusually extensive and extremely carefully evaluated body of material, the pathological-anatomic and histologic foundation of one of the most important diseases of the brain is secured and expanded in a way from which every future work on this difficult topic will have to proceed."

The test lecture took place on July 23, 1904, at 11:30 A.M. in the lecture hall of the psychiatric clinic. The topic was announced as "Hysterical Mental Disorders," so the somaticist Alzheimer became for a short time a "psychicist." He thus followed a contemporary trend: It had not escaped his attention that in 1900 neurologist Sigmund Freud had published *The Interpretation of Dreams*.

Freud deliberately chose the year 1900 as the date of his book's appearance because he was sure that he had created an epoch-making work. In his book Freud presents, first and foremost, the results of the self-analysis to which he had subjected himself in a concentrated way since the summer of 1895.

The dean's office expressed its positive views on Alzheimer's work to the academic senate on the day of the lecture: "The content of his lecture was well-thought-out and clear, and its form was thoroughly satisfactory.

Dr. Alzheimer carried out the defense of his theses with great composure and decided mastery of the subject."

On August 10, 1904, the dean's office received the report from the senate that Alois Alzheimer had been named to the position of privatdozent by ministerial decree; no less a personage than Prince Regent Luitpold had approved it. With that Dr. Alzheimer became a member of the medical faculty of the Royal Ludwig-Maximilian University in Munich.

The scientific work that brought him the *venia legendi* does not address the clinical picture that later made him famous; this is not surprising because at that time the picture seldom appeared. The *Habilitation* has far more to do with a disease whose victims filled the mental asylums of Alzheimer's times: dementia paralytica or general paresis, progressive "softening" of the brain.

"It refers to a progressive imbecility with a great many signs of irritation and paresis" is how Kraepelin expressed it in 1904 in the seventh edition of his *Textbook for Students and Doctors*. It was not known at the time that this condition was a late consequence of syphilis. There was therefore a substantial need for research, driven by the high admission numbers in the asylums.

At the time of Alzheimer's *Habilitation*, about a third of the inmates of psychiatric institutions suffered from tertiary syphilis, and the trend was for that proportion to increase, especially in the big cities. The numbers in Munich and Berlin ranged from 36 percent of the male paretics in Munich to 45.6 percent in Berlin's Charité.

The admission numbers were twice as high in the cities as in predominantly rural environments. Kraepelin reported that "in individual countries, such as Iceland, general paresis is almost unknown; it has spread significantly among the Negroes of North America only in the last decade." Men were affected approximately two and a half times as often as women. The average duration of the disease was thirty-three months for men, forty-seven for women, although the numbers varied widely.

Alzheimer was among those who believed that a connection between paresis and syphilis was probable in approximately 70 percent of the congenital cases, or juvenile general paresis. Other clinicians held a hereditary disposition responsible, and alcohol abuse was also regarded as a cause. Nevertheless, the anatomic findings were the same as those in adult paresis.

Kraepelin continued,

Single people appear to be more threatened than married; young female paretics are strikingly often prostitutes, and paretic women are, in many cases, childless. Not infrequently one observes that both members of a married couple simultaneously, or one shortly after the other, become paretic or tabetic [afflicted with atrophy of the spinal cord].

Among the professions, military officers, salespeople, firefighters, and railway officials are represented in large numbers, whereas Catholic clergy very rarely become paretic. Among patients from the clergy Caboureau found that only 1.9 percent were paretic, in contrast to the general average of 17.5 percent. Among 2000 paretics, Von Krafft-Ebing also saw not a single member of the Catholic clergy but up to 90 percent paretics among mentally ill officers.

Syphilis was considered first among the causes of general paresis: "My own records show, in agreement with von Gudden's experiences at the Charité, syphilis as a certainty in 34 percent of the cases of men," wrote Kraepelin;

Seen as a whole, many points of general predisposition, in particular the differences between city and country, the rarity of paresis among women of the better classes and among Catholic clergy, its frequency among officers, businesspeople, and prostitutes, and the appearance of paretic married couples and siblings with great probability, are interpreted as indicating that a strong correlation exists between paresis and syphilis. This point of view is made uncertain by the opinion of the majority of French psychiatrists, who deny the causal importance of syphilis for paresis and emphasize alcohol abuse instead.[17]

The issue was clarified in 1917, when Oswald Bumke published his *Textbook of Mental Illnesses*: "Today we no longer need to go into the now historical dispute as to whether paresis is always determined by syphilis. All of the individual data point in this direction: that the illness appears more frequently in men than in women and is more widespread in certain professions than others, that it can be found in cases of virgo intacta only when an extragenital syphilis can be proven, and in children only when the parents can be proven syphilitic, and that it has at certain times been absent from entire peoples. All of these experiences can today be reduced to a formula: Paresis can emerge only where there is syphilis."[18]

Alzheimer approached the problem of general paresis especially thoroughly in his work: "All cases of mental disorder that appeared for autopsy in the course of my work at the Municipal Mental Asylum at Frankfurt in the last seven years were tested histologically. That makes 320 cases. The number of observations may well be large enough that chance occurrences in the tissue findings can be recognized as such, the possibilities and limits of deviation can be determined, and all of the characteristics of paresis discovered."

Still more important, and a trademark of his work, is the last paragraph of his introduction: "The results of these investigations will be a gauge of the extent to which pathological histology can prove itself to be of use for clinical psychiatry."

Alzheimer thus proclaimed his intention to study psychiatric symptoms with the microscope. He wanted to drive research on the causes of illness forward and place the subject on a solid, organic foundation, as it was in other fields of medicine.

What Alzheimer achieved in Frankfurt from 1888 to 1903 is inconceivable today: He examined all paretic patients for the *Habilitation* thesis himself, carrying out the autopsies and evaluating the brains, macroscopically and microscopically, with his own hands.

Along with co-worker Eva Schmidt, Alzheimer personally made and signed all fourteen illustrations in the *Habilitation* thesis, which should be regarded as works of art. In the thesis Alzheimer describes twenty-six cases in detail; the corresponding case histories contain extensive dialogues that Alzheimer conducted with his patients.

One example of these is the case of the forty-six-year-old master butcher I.D., who was admitted on August 21, 1901, with a suspected diagnosis of general paresis. I.D. was very agitated and fearful and constantly wanted to go outside. He perspired heavily and had a strong tremor of the hands, searched for the door in odd places, and in his behavior resembled someone suffering a delirium.

Under closer observation, however, Alzheimer detected that he could not speak properly; he showed no understanding of the questions directed to him and had only a few words at his disposal, which he repeated constantly: "Yes, what is then, what is then, the hunters, the hunters."

Alzheimer posed questions relentlessly and tested thoroughly. The patient correctly identified individual objects that were held in front of him:

"Ten-pfennig piece?"

"Tenner."

"Twenty-pfennig piece?"

"Twentier."

"Mark piece?"

"That is a mark, money."

"Pencil?"

"Pencil."

"Safety pin?"

He looked at the pin and fiddled with it. "That is a pincenel, right?" He briefly looked up and regarded Alzheimer's pince-nez with a mischievous expression.

Alzheimer continued: "Bread roll?"

"Bread roll."

"What is your name?"

"Hm, yes."

"Where are you?"

"Yes."

"How old are you?"

"Yes."

"Stick out your tongue!"

"Yes, yes."

"Stick your hand out!"

"Yes, yes, the first ball, pass ball."

"How are you?"

"Yes, I am saying yes."

Alzheimer examined the patient and immediately discovered typical signs of a progressive paresis: narrow, unequal pupils, both of which remained fixed and unresponsive to light. (Alzheimer was checking for a form of reflex iridoplegia known as Argyll Robertson pupil, after a Scottish ophthalmologist.) The patellar reflex could not be induced.

According to the file, Alzheimer saw his patient every day. On August 23, 1901, he put a newspaper in the patient's hand, whereupon the patient at first turned away, irritated, but then correctly read the title: "*Generalanzieger* No. 187, Frankfurt am Main, Sunday, August 12, 1900." He also read the smaller print fluently but then began again: "I can't read, I can fifty-four, I have away, I am in my fiftieth year, in front I am a wound, I reading indeed, I don't want to any more."

The patient died on January 16, 1902, after showing a rapid decline in strength in the final weeks. Alzheimer performed the autopsy himself and confirmed his clinical diagnosis:

> The assumption of the admitting colleague, that this was a case of a traumatic psychosis in consequence of a bleeding in the brain, . . . could not be excluded at the time of admission. But the first, more precise examination already produced findings that guaranteed the diagnosis of paresis and indicated an already widespread disease: absence of the patellar reflex and reflex iridoplegia, to which were soon added paralytic disturbances of speech and writing.

At the conclusion of the case description he remarked, "In view of the localization of the paretic illness we have here a case of the most serious disease of the temporal and parietal lobes, with limited involvement of the frontal lobe and central gyri."

Alzheimer impressively described the mental disintegration of general paresis:

> The damage attaches to all capacities. Memory and judgment, feeling and intention suffer from the outset. The sick person becomes increasingly detached from the outside world because he becomes more and more incapable both of understanding the impressions made by his environment and of bringing in relation to his own personality the little that he still absorbs. He soon also loses any ability to observe and to judge his own self.
>
> Thus he soon loses all understanding of his condition and either falls into a dumb euphoria, which presents a harsh contrast to his actual situation, or he becomes an uncritical victim, susceptible to every influence and to intermittent illusions. His memory be-

comes dull, his old memories and experiences are no longer discernible and disintegrate, his interests melt together. Nothing is left of his earlier personality.

Finally he sits there in a stupor, utterly without mental stirring; perhaps one sees him still betray a few animal cravings while eating. Along with the mental disintegration gradually accumulate, in rapidly increasing severity and multiplicity, signs of paresis, in part caused by the progressive destruction of the cerebral cortex, in part conditioned by changes in tissue that have taken place in deeper parts of the brain and in the spinal cord.

In his *Habilitation* thesis Alzheimer had undoubtedly established a milestone in the history of clinical psychiatry. All modesty aside, he appeared well aware of the implications of his work: "The question of whether a case is one of paresis will hardly ever have to remain open after a satisfactory histologic examination. Clinical psychiatry thereby acquires an aid that other branches of medicine have already made successful use of for a long time."

In his one-page summary of his *Habilitation* thesis, Alzheimer arrived, as he did so often, at the knowledge that general paresis is a histologically distinct disease. The last sentence was also typical of him: "However, the entire examination should demonstrate only that pathological histology is a useful complementary science to psychiatry." At the end of his *Habilitation* thesis he thanked his former boss, director Sioli, for allowing him to use the case histories and the examination material.

A year after Alzheimer's *Habilitation* thesis, on March 3, 1905, an important discovery was made: German zoologist Fritz Schaudinn, with his colleague Erich Hoffmann, found the syphilis pathogen. At first they called it *Spirochaeta pallida* and later *Treponema pallidum*.

In 1906 Berlin bacteriologist August von Wassermann, director of the unit for experimental therapy and serum research at the Royal Institute for Infectious Diseases in Berlin, together with dermatologist Albert Neisser, announced a sensational success. He published in the *Deutschen Medizinischen Wochenschrift* (*German Medical Weekly*) a method by which syphilis could be diagnosed definitively. Syphilis and its late forms, general paresis and *Tabes dorsalis* (wasting of the spinal cord), could thus be diagnosed without the need for autopsy and ensuing microscopic examination.

From 1907 on the Munich clinic had a laboratory for the serodiagnosis of syphilis, directed by Felix Plaut. Wassermann's Berlin laboratory was Plaut's model; earlier, Kraepelin had sent Plaut to Berlin to conduct experiments, predominantly with cerebrospinal fluid from paretic patients and with blood serums. The serodiagnostic laboratory in Munich soon was just as famous as the one in Berlin, and many colleagues from Germany and beyond came to Nussbaumstrasse to learn the new examination methods.

Initially syphilis was treated with mercury, first in the form of an ointment, later as an injection. However, this therapy had severe effects on the kidneys and nerves. Only in 1910 was a treatment developed that was substantially more effective than mercury, when Paul Ehrlich and Sahatschiro Hata developed arsphenamine (also called Salvarsan).

After his epoch-making work on general paresis, Alzheimer turned more intensively to the psychoses and dementias.

## Family Life

"That father chose an apartment precisely on Rükertstrasse was no accident. For one, it was just a few minutes' walk from the clinic; also, he felt himself quasi-magically attracted to such houses." The houses Alzheimer's son, Hans, spoke of were the generous bourgeois homes built at the end of the nineteenth century in the *Gründerzeit* style.

As little as he was at home, Alzheimer loved life with his children. At that time fathers were considered unapproachable authority figures, strict and feared, especially when a child failed in some way. Alois Alzheimer did not conform at all to the stereotype of his time: He was kind and lenient and tolerated slip-ups with humor.

He wanted to inspire his children with his passion for nature, and so he taught them to observe closely and thus to learn new things. His son, Hans, recounts,

> Father thought it quite important for us children always to have animals around us and also to learn early on to care for them. So we had rabbits, guinea pigs, and fish in the garden and in the apartment. He even brought a young fox home, but it immediately rejected the dog hut and took to its heels.

Once he carefully put on the floor a big, mysteriously covered basket. Through the wickerwork of the basket I saw two big yellow eyes and heard some peculiar croaking. My father explained that it was an owl that he had caught in the park. He raised the cover and out hopped the big bird, which in the next moment went and sat on the curtain. Family members must have protested against the new tenant, because the next day the owl had already vanished; father had let it out in the park.

Already as a small child Hans received a botanist's specimen box and a butterfly net, with which he caught his booty and proudly presented it to his father. When he found a rare moth or an unknown beetle, he could impress his father with it because he was constantly in search of such rarities.

Father and son also went exploring together and systematically collected beetles, moths, and butterflies, which they then anesthetized with ether, killed, and pinned in display boxes. The German and Latin name of each arthropod stood beneath it in small handwriting. Exotic butterfly pupae, which Hans received for Christmas in 1904, were the highlight of this "research."

With amazement he watched the fairytale-like process by which giant, gloriously colorful, shimmering butterflies hatched out of the bland pupae. Nevertheless, they ultimately ended up in a glass display case and over the years were admired again and again.

Another time Hans discovered a dead shrew, which his father took from him and put in an anthill. After a while the two of them dug up the skeleton, which had been stripped bare by the ants, and then Alzheimer explained to his son that the shrew was not a rodent but a small predator, as one could see from the animal's teeth.

Soon after the move to Munich, the house on Wesslinger Lake became a genuine Eldorado for the children. They could let off steam there, and from that time on Alzheimer spent many weekends at the house with his family. One of his granddaughters still lives in this idyllic home today. Hans tells the story of how Alois Alzheimer surprised the family with the purchase of this house at Christmas in 1904:

The family celebrated Christmases in Rückertstrasse in Munich. On the first day of the holiday papa said, "All right, now we'll go

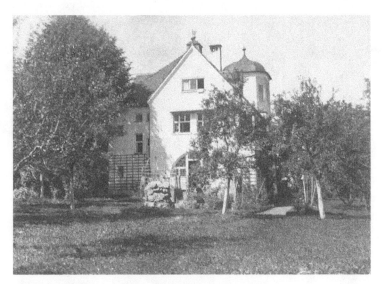

FIGURE 5.5  *The vacation house in Wessling, near Munich*

to Wessling." "To Wessling, now, in winter?" the children wondered. Before this they had only been able to spend summer vaca-
tions there. So they took the steam train to Wessling and trudged
about in the snow around the frozen lake. But where was father taking them? He knocked on a big door. Nothing happened. He stuck
his hand in his trouser pocket and pulled out a big key. "Let's see
whether this fits!" To everyone's great surprise, it did.

The gate opened, squeaking. Behind it, in a small stand of
beech trees, lay moss-covered stone steps, and at the top, in bright
light—there stood the house! A wonderful house! This is what father had given the children for Christmas. It lies somewhat elevated, directly on the lake. In the farmhouse parlor a fire crackled
in a large, green-tiled stove. To our joy, there was a lot to explore:
the many rooms and the big garden. A hill passed through the garden, and at the top stood an alpine hut; through the back garden
gate one could get to the forest, through the front the banks of the
lake, where there was also a boathouse.

The house could not be compared with other domiciles because a benevolent house spirit moved in with the family, and this
had the effect of making everyone feel happy and at home there. It
was an Alzheimer house and has remained so today.

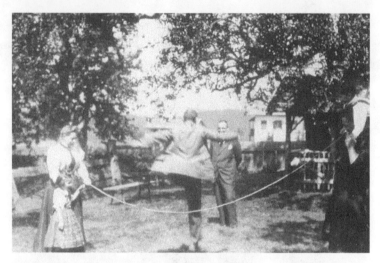

FIGURE 5.6 *Alzheimer jumping rope*

The photographs showing Alzheimer with his family and friends in front of his house on the lake or at the coffee table do not give the impression that this gigantic man is an academic. His erect posture has something military about it, although his entire manner, his calm and natural spirit, radiates sympathy and trust. He loved comfort and was not averse to life's pleasures, which found foremost expression in his predilection for good cigars. He had a great sense of humor, although in contrast to his student years, when he was boisterous, he found noisy conviviality unpleasant. Although he had no understanding of music, now and then he picked up a guitar and strummed it; he had little interest in any other arts and was largely indifferent to them, nor did he enjoy imaginary play and daydreaming. At this time, he was as affable as ever, although over the years the tension of professional life cost him a great deal of his cheerfulness and liveliness.

His supreme ease also expressed itself in the composed way with which he dealt with extraordinary situations. Hans reports on a break-in at Wessling:

> I slunk back home with bad grades—what would father say? But my little sister Maria met me, very excited, because our house in Wessling had been broken into—fine by me, because now no one was going to ask me about my grades.
>
> Father sat at his writing desk, reading through the insurance

policies, and said that Wessling was well insured. He shook his head: How was that possible, with a good caretaker, two dogs, whose kennels were at the house, bars, locks, and bolts—of course—everything was in order! The ladies feared for linen, jewelry, and silver, and we were all prepared for the worst. Father proposed an immediate expedition to Wessling. Awaiting us there was an embarrassed caretaker: He said that he had heard a rustling yesterday and then nothing until the dogs barked at 2 o'clock, but then it had been quiet again.

As it turned out, the dogs had been bribed with bones, so the thieves could easily get into the house through the windows above the dog kennels. The linen was gone, hangers and all, and everything was a mess. Instead of father's loden hat a strange, dirty cap hung on the hook, and he was also missing a suit and shoes. After that, the fourteen-year-old dachshund was found to be too old and given to a neighbor, and a new dog had to be brought in. Father's choice was a Doberman from the breeding kennels in Apolda. A telegram was immediately dispatched. The patrolman came and wrote the list of losses in his notebook and said that he knew the delinquents and would undoubtedly catch them. On this particular day father did not ask about my grades.

Alois Alzheimer's generosity was almost limitless. When his thirteen-year-old daughter once asked him, "Papa, when I have big debts one day, what will you do then?" he answered laconically, "Pay!" He bought his brother Eduard, after the completion of his pharmacy studies, the Elisabeth Pharmacy in Munich-Schwabing. The household on Wessling Lake was run just as openly and generously and soon became a meeting place for all the siblings.

Alzheimer was happy to have his siblings and their children around him. Only for Aunt Malchen, Alfred's wife, Amalie, was his affection limited because she talked too much for his liking. He tolerated her, but sometimes he would have preferred to be rid of her; then he would curse her with the pidgin Latin sentence "Et libera nos a Malo!" (actually, "and liberate us from evil").

Aunt Anna, the wife of his older brother, Karl, was not spared either. She was addressed as "Mrs. *Geheimrat*" (privy councillor) because she was

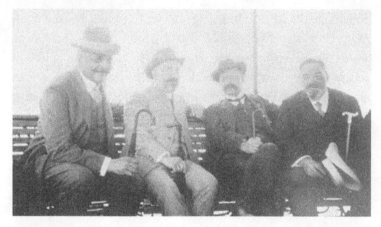

FIGURE 5.7 *Alzheimer, Kraepelin, Gaupp, and Nissl during an excursion on Lake Starnberg*

very prim. During a Shrovetide carnival he tried everything he could to make her laugh. As Hans later recounted, "He dressed himself up as a ballerina and forced his stately legs into a pink cotton leotard, fastened a tutu about himself, tried out some graceful contortions and blew kisses to aunt Anna. Did she laugh, or was she shocked?"

Apart from Alzheimer's siblings, many of his medical colleagues also passed through the house in Wessling, undertaking excursions together. Kraepelin described these tours in his memoirs:

> So it happened that we never went beyond the region of the Isar Valley and the Starnberg and Ammer lakes. At first I only went into the mountains once, when I made a short excursion up the Schachen and from there over the Walchen Lake and Herzogstand. Later I tried to spend a few Sundays every summer in the mountains. In winter I regularly went tobogganing once or twice, mostly on the Herzogstand.

On one of these tours photographs were taken that show Alzheimer with Kraepelin, Gaupp, and Nissl. A picture from 1908 is especially impressive: Alzheimer, Kraepelin, Gaupp, and Nissl in a cheerful mood during a boat ride on Starnberg Lake.

According to Kraepelin, such trips were more the exception than the rule. He often tried to draw the inexhaustible scientist away from his workplace:

At my insistence he forced himself in the late evening hours to go for a short walk through the streets; he knew hardly any other form of relaxation. It was nearly impossible to get him to take a long vacation; after a short time he would be back, in order not to have to leave this or that work unfinished. He always found excuses to defer rest until later.

Only in later years did he get himself a home in the country that offered him the welcome opportunity to work in the garden and to pursue his botanic hobbies. It was also possible for me to tempt him into climbing a mountain; this was difficult for him because he thought he had no time for physical activity.

In the clinic, despite his devotion to his work and his seriousness, he was receptive to all sorts of jokes and showed a good sense of humor, as one of the granddaughters recalls:

It was Fashing [carnival] in the Nussbaumstrasse clinic in Munich. A poor peddler arrived, completely unexpectedly, with a sales tray full of toys hanging around his neck, offering his wares for sale. This didn't go over well: He was angrily prevented from plying his trade and threatened that Prof. Alzheimer would be brought in, and he would show him a thing or two. "That is not necessary," said the peddler mischievously and took off his disguise. Everyone had to laugh. The professor as peddler! He distributed the toys to the young patients. Yes, gift-giving always gave him great joy.

### In the Anatomy Laboratory

Alzheimer followed Kraepelin to Munich principally because, as his boss had promised him, extensive opportunities for experimentation and corresponding laboratory rooms for his cerebro-pathological and histopathological research would available to him there. Kraepelin wrote, "After Nissl was already, after a short time, called to the chair at Heidelberg, the task fell to Alzheimer alone of setting up the Munich clinic's splendid anatomic work rooms and filling them with life."

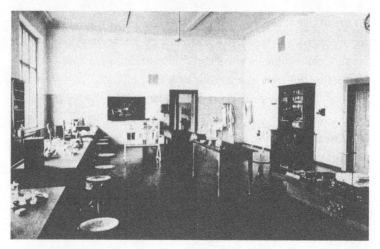

FIGURE 5.8 *Microscopy laboratory in the Munich clinic*

As an experienced researcher, Alzheimer knew exactly what equipment was needed. After a few weeks everything was in its place, and he could begin his work. The work room contained numerous tables but was large enough to allow experimenters to move about freely. Alzheimer had a number of work tables installed at the glass facades, and the microscopes stood there, in front of adjustable stools.

Meanwhile, the camera lucida, with which slide preparations could be drawn directly, had also been installed. The cabinets were filled with reagents. At the end of the room stood a shelf on castors, on which stood buckets containing the fluids needed to prepare slides. Two wall telephones were also available, with which results could be given directly to the treating doctor.

Alzheimer spent many hours in his lab, taking special pleasure in patiently explaining histopathological sections to his students. Karl Kleist, Emil Sioli's successor in Frankfurt, who worked with Alzheimer in the winter semester of 1908–09, conveyed his impressions of the laboratory:

His large laboratory was filled with students from all corners of the earth, and Alzheimer taught every single one inexhaustibly, devotedly, selflessly, without ever letting the strain show. Every morning and every afternoon—and later—he came into the laboratory and went from work station to work station, taught us to

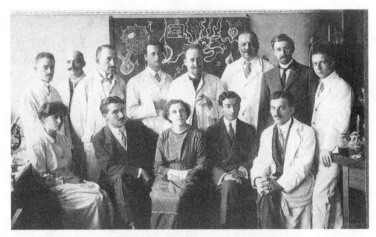

FIGURE 5.9  *Guest doctors in the anatomy laboratory: top row from left: F. Lotmar, unknown, St. Rosental, Allers (?), unknown, Alzheimer, N. Achucarro, F. H. Levy; bottom row from left: Mrs. Grombach, U. Cerletti, unknown, F. Bonfiglio, G. Perusini*

see every detail in the microscopic image, to recognize its characteristics and to draw conclusions from it. If the co-workers came back to the lab at 3 o'clock, he had been there since 2 o'clock. He loved this hour in which he was undisturbed.[19]

Among these students were many researchers who later gained prestige in their fields: N. Achucarro from Spain, Francesco Bonfiglio from Italy, and Louis Casamajor from the United States.

In 1908 Bonfiglio published on a case of presenile dementia that aroused Kraepelin's interest. Ugo Cerletti, from Italy, became world famous in 1938 when he, together with L. Bini, used electrical shocks to produce convulsions in people for the first time, beginning the era of electroconvulsive therapy; in 1936 he became director of the Clinica delle Malattie Nervose e Mentali in Rome.

Hans Gerhard Creutzfeldt and Alfons Jakob also became world renowned through the illness later named after them, Creutzfeldt–Jakob disease, which was later included among the slow virus infections. This illness could be passed on to chimpanzees, who became ill after an incubation period of a year; in 1968 Daniel Gajdusek received the Nobel prize in medicine for this discovery.

The influenza pandemic that spread after World War I was named after Constantin von Economo, Baron of San Serff, who discovered a "sleep
steering center" in the midbrain. F. Lotmar came from Switzerland and ran
the chemistry laboratory. Merzbacher–Pelizaeus disease, or familial cen-
trolobar sclerosis, was named after Ludwig Merzbacher, who first worked
in Tübingen and later in Buenos Aires. The Lewy bodies, which play a role
in Parkinson's disease, were named after Frederic H. Lewy.

Gaetano Perusini warrants special emphasis: He worked with Alzheimer a great deal and also published with him. In 1909 he published extensively on the famous case of Auguste D., contributing to the spread of
the designation *Alzheimer's*.

Perusini resembled Alzheimer in many respects: Both came from good
homes, both were financially independent (Perusini through inheritance,
Alzheimer through marriage), and both had an insatiable interest in neuropathology. Perusini's family came from Cormóns in Friaul, which at that
time belonged to the Austro-Hungarian Empire. The family had excellent
connections to high nobility: Perusini's mother was a close friend of the
Hapsburgs, and they owned the castle Rocca Bernarda in Cormóns. Perusini was born in 1879, was raised by a governess, and spoke fluent German. He worked in Alzheimer's laboratory until 1912.[20]

Coincidentally, the dates of their deaths also are very close: Perusini
died at just thirty-six on December 8, 1915, a week before Alois Alzheimer,
of a fatal injury sustained in World War I during an attempt to help a
wounded soldier.

With his great pedagogical skill Alzheimer thus left his mark on a new
generation of neuropathologists. The otherwise reserved Kraepelin praised
him for it: "It was therefore obvious that within a short time the work sta-
tions were filled with competent researchers from all corners of the earth
and that under his tireless leadership and stimulus a series of valuable
works emerged."

Alzheimer's trademark soon became his omnipresent cigar, which,
caught up in the enthusiasm of his explanations, he often left burning at the
work station of one of his students, so that every evening the laboratory
was shrouded in a haze from burnt-down cigars.

The clinic's funding did not begin to cover the many tasks and expen-
sive methods to which Alzheimer and his co-workers devoted themselves
in the anatomy laboratory. In his well-known generosity Alzheimer not

only declined a salary but also paid the majority of the costs incurred in his laboratory, such as the preparation of drawings and photographs, the salaries of assistant personnel, and the acquisition of a diverse collection of supplies and equipment.

"Despite everything," wrote Kraepelin, "he was a long way from setting boundaries on his activity in the anatomy laboratory. With the unshakable loyalty and dependability that characterized him, he supported me devotedly in the difficult initial establishment of the clinic as well as in smoothing out the internal friction that arose here and there and in the general supervision of the medical service. The unconditional trust that everyone felt for him and his calm objectivity helped to smooth out conflicts and resolve difficulties so that he imperceptibly became the cornerstone of the entire clinical operation."

The extent to which Alzheimer valued his research is also illustrated by the equanimity with which he coped with not being in the spotlight. The anatomic results and the histologic sections were demonstrated during Kraepelin's lectures, at which Alzheimer was almost always present. Only rarely did he stand in for his boss and give the lecture himself, and then, "he spoke excellently, without any rhetoric but filled with practical enthusiasm. As difficult as the material was that he lectured on to an often inexpert audience, he always succeeded in making it gripping and in giving the audience an insight into his research."[21]

The limited attention Kraepelin gave to Alzheimer's work did not bother Alzheimer much. The great teacher of psychiatry seldom went up to the fourth floor of the anatomy laboratory. Adele Grombach, who worked as Alzheimer's technical assistant and later at the Research Institute under Alzheimer's successor, Spielmeyer, introducing co-workers and guests to neurohistologic techniques until the end of World War II, recounts how Kraepelin appeared there one day:

He strode through the large rooms and looked at everything with interest. As he left the laboratory again, everyone looked at him expectantly: "Yes, yes, the anatomical mills grind very slowly!" remarked the central opinion-maker in German psychiatry. He gave praise very rarely, and he knew that the remark he had just made would stir up still further the colleagues' enthusiasm for work.[22]

Afterwards, Kraepelin left the laboratory and, according to Adele Grombach, was seen only a few times after that.

## Responsibility as Chief Physician

Alzheimer's confidence and standing at the clinic were so strong that Kraepelin's application on September 6, 1906, to propose him as chief physician and to confer upon him the right to deputize in overseeing the work of the board, including signing receipts, did not set off a storm of excitement in Alzheimer because he would thereby have to give up some of his independence. Kraepelin described it thus:

> In 1906 my chief physician at that time, Gaupp, was appointed to a full professorship in Tübingen. The choice of an appropriate successor gave me great difficulties. I did not know any more appropriate and to me more welcome person than my loyal co-worker Alzheimer. On a trip that we undertook together to the Idiot Asylum in Eckberg, I asked him to take over the position of chief physician at least temporarily. It was a great sacrifice that I was asking of him because he would have to give up the complete freedom of scientific work that he enjoyed, and he was not a man to take duties lightly once he had assumed them. With a heavy heart, and after a long struggle, he agreed to it under the condition that after a fitting time he could step down again.[22]

Thus on October 25, 1906, Alzheimer became leading chief physician under Kraepelin and successor to Robert Gaupp, who later became known primarily for the Wagner case, a case study that simultaneously represented a contribution to the theory of paranoia. The Wagner case, along with Freud's Anna O. and Alzheimer's Auguste D., is one of the best-known case histories in psychiatry.

As chief physician Alzheimer also received an income: In 1908 he earned a salary of 2700 marks per annum, which consisted of a base salary of 2280 marks, a salary bonus, and a personal bonus of 60 marks. In 1909 his salary was raised to 3000 marks.

In addition to his activity as a researcher and chief physician, Alzheimer dedicated himself to teaching students and learned that the burden of clinical duties and teaching, of meetings and examinations, would make it increasingly difficult for him to focus his attention on scientific questions. As a consequence, Kraepelin in particular had little time to occupy himself with the questions of experimental psychology.

In experimental psychology, Kraepelin became a bestower of names: Kraepelin's arithmetic test, which measures fatigue and drive, is named after him.

Under the increasing workload it was no wonder that Kraepelin bemoaned his situation: "All attempts to get the obstructive difficulties under control came to nothing, and I had to console myself with the hope that perhaps at the end of my career, when the burden of the office would be taken from me, I would be able to return to my old interests."

Both Kraepelin and Alzheimer held two-hour afternoon lectures on psychiatry twice a week, during which they presented five or six patients in a row each time. It turned out that this division of time allowed a better explanation of the clinical picture than did the one-hour lectures. Kraepelin retained the two-hour schedule when he later shifted the clinical lecture to midday, from 11 A.M. to 1 P.M. It was their goal during the semester to teach the students essential psychiatric knowledge through practical learning.

The lectures usually began with an easily understood illness such as melancholia. Kraepelin then developed through the presentation of manic patients the concept of manic–depressive insanity and then moved on to different clinical pictures such as dementia praecox—that is, schizophrenia—and general paresis, and then concluded with the causally transparent forms such as alcoholism and morphine addiction.

Alzheimer was closely involved in the lectures on the treatment of general paresis and arteriosclerotic, senile, and syphilitic brain diseases, and he often presented slides.

Kraepelin and Alzheimer constantly maintained lists of cases appropriate for teaching purposes, selected the appropriate patients before the lectures, and updated their index cards, which they used for their later statistical evaluations. They thereby saved a lot of time because processing case histories took less time than teaching itself. Kraepelin's lectures, at which

Alzheimer was an almost constant presence, were of a high quality and were regularly attended by about 200 listeners.

In the lectures Alzheimer and Kraepelin particularly liked to use modern aids such as cinematography. To this end they set up a room with nine lamps that could be illuminated to make cinematographic pictures. Over the years a large number of films showing epileptic, hysterical, and paralytic attacks were developed in this way.

Furthermore, manic and catatonic (that is, motor-disturbed) states of excitement and stereotypies (repetitive behaviors), idiotic movements, delirious behavior, and peripatetic disorders of all kinds were recorded and reproduced during lectures.

At the same time, Alzheimer also cultivated a large collection of slides that showed mainly microscopic changes in the most important diseases of the cerebral cortex. Kraepelin wrote,

> The largest lecture undertaking that we brought to life, however, was a series of continuing education courses for specialist colleagues held for years. They emerged out of the desire to give to all who wanted to perfect themselves in our science an overview of the most recent state of our knowledge in the most diverse branches in the brief time of eight weeks.
>
> Apart from the clinical presentations that I arranged, which stood in the center of the course, Alzheimer gave an overview of the pathological anatomy of the psychoses, and Brodmann, who had come from Tübingen, reported on the topographic histology of the cerebral cortex. Liepmann from Berlin and von Monakow from Zürich spoke alternately on questions of localization, Rüdin on hereditary and degeneration theory, Blaut on serology, Allers on metabolic examinations, and I offered a short sketch of clinical experimental psychology. The attendance at this course was very satisfying and consisted of around forty to fifty participants, among which, however, foreigners tended to predominate.[24]

Word had gotten around throughout Germany and Europe that the clinicians Kraepelin and Alzheimer were the premier clinical neuropathologists. Brain pathology assumed a central position in the field, and more and more international researchers made their way to Alzheimer's laboratory.

In addition to his duties as teacher, chief physician Alzheimer often had to stand in for Kraepelin, especially when Kraepelin, as was often the case, went on trips or retreated to his country house in Pollenza on Lago Maggiore to work on his textbooks. From 1907 to 1909 Alzheimer stood in for his director six times in all, once for eight weeks.

During one of these periods an incident took place at the clinic. A mentally disturbed female patient committed suicide in an unobserved moment by pouring spirits over herself and then setting herself on fire. Alzheimer wrote an extensive report, which he sent to the Royal State Ministry for Internal, Church, and School Matters, and said in conclusion,

> This is obviously a case of the nurse's gross negligence as well as a breach of duty on the part of the house maid, both of whom acted against constantly repeated instructions not to leave patients alone. This had been especially impressed upon the nurse in direct relation to this particular patient on the day before. We have therefore had to make a report to the Royal Police headquarters.[25]

## The Fruits of Labor

Alzheimer had arrived in Munich in the fall of 1903. In 1904 the old enthusiasm for congresses and publication seized him again.

In Frankfurt, under Sioli, his scientific focal point had been the clearly defined diseases of the brain, the so-called exogenous psychoses with inflammatory, vascular-conditioned, and neurodegenerative brain diseases. In Munich his focus became the investigation of endogenous psychoses and an engagement with Kraepelin's theory of disease.

Alzheimer posed himself this challenge and applied his histopathological methods to patients with schizophrenia and manic—depressive disease, or bipolar disorder.

He performed this work in addition to his duties as chief physician and deputy director of a large university clinic. Alzheimer clearly understood that in view of the imminent understanding about general paresis—syphilis would soon be recognized as its cause—he had to find another focal point for his research. There was one field that he never lost sight of: presenile dementia and its key case, that of Auguste D.

His 1904 lecture in Baden-Baden in 1904, "Alcoholic Delirium Magnans," reflected Alzheimer's activities in Frankfurt, where with his usual diligence he had examined 160 patients with delirium. In Baden-Baden he described three cases in detail. Febrile alcoholic delirium Magnans, later called delirium tremens, was accompanied by a strong tremor, drowsiness, excessive perspiration, and an elevated temperature. Jacques Joseph-Valentin Magnan (1835–1916) was head of the admissions unit at the Hospital Sainte-Anne in Paris and a recognized expert on delirium, and in 1874 he wrote the textbook on alcoholism.

As exciting as ever, Alzheimer held forth,

My three cases were strong men between the ages of thirty and forty, and were all schnapps drinkers. In the families of my patients cases of delirium occurred frequently. The deliria of my patients began with a great restlessness, a so-called delirium of activity, hallucinations, disorientation in relation to the environment, violent tremors, and excessive outbreaks of perspiration. The mood was peculiarly irritable and gruff.

After the beginning of the delirious symptoms, each of my patients had an epileptic seizure, and shortly thereafter a noticeable fever appeared in which I could measure temperatures of 39.4, 39.6, and even 40 degrees Celsius. The first patient died five, the second eight, and the last fourteen hours after the beginning of the symptoms of delirium. Shortly before decease I measured extremely high temperatures of 39.4, 40.1, and even 41.8 degrees Celsius.

Because Alzheimer had performed the autopsies on these patients, he could report in Baden-Baden what everybody already expected: "Along with the sort of results one could have found with chronic alcoholism, especially seriously diseased conditions and symptoms of decay in the ganglial cells also appeared." Then Alzheimer turned to the board on which his slides were projected: "Growth processes could be seen on the glial cells. In the cortex I found numerous tiny hemorrhages and an especially serious degeneration of the capillaries. Nowhere could a trace of an inflammatory process be seen."

He thus concluded his lecture: "In my opinion there is, of course, a *delirium alcoholicum febrile*. It does not always pass into recovery or into

the Korsakov symptom complex [a combination of disorientation, memory disturbance, and the mixing up of sounds in words] but rather it can,
conditioned by further complicating diseases and by the severity of the disease processes thus conditioned, lead to death, as seen in my three cases."[26]

Alzheimer's colleagues applauded him with a loud knocking on the
desks; questions about the therapy dominated the lively discussion that
followed.

According to the prevailing opinion, opium achieved "the best and
most secure service. . . . Next to that, one prescribed, as soon as any signs
of cardiac weakness were apparent, large doses of cognac. Eventually cam-
phor injections and cold dousings are considered. Outside the asylum,
when faced with states of intense agitation during which an isolation room
cannot be improvised, one injects hyoscine; the highest initial dosage is
measured in these cases at 0.6 milligrams. Nutrition requires the most precise control."[27]

The publication "A Few Points About the Anatomic Foundations of
Idiocy," which appeared in 1904 in the renowned *Zentralblatt für Nervenheilkunde und Psychiatrie* (*Central Journal of Neurology and Psychiatry*), confirmed Alzheimer's versatility and his broad clinical interests.[28] Alzheimer
classified idiocy among the dementias acquired during or shortly after birth
and in early adolescence.

> Already in the macroscopic observation of the idiot's brain one
> sees a series of distinct findings that belong more or less exclu-
> sively to idiocy, such as microencephaly and macroencephaly
> (large and small brains), microgyria and macrogyria (gyri that are
> too large or too small), porencephaly, in this case crater-shaped
> collections on the surface of the brain, and finally hydrocephalus,
> that is, water on the brain.

Afterward he mentioned amaurotic idiocy, a lipometabolic disorder
that is accompanied by psychomotor retardation, increasing visual disturbances, and pareses. Alzheimer was a recognized specialist in this clinical picture because he had examined thirty cases of it in Frankfurt. The
first symptoms of the disease usually appeared within the first year of life.
After a few months the disease led to death. The child who until that
point had developed well forgot how to play, eat, and sit and began to

drool, swallowed with difficulty, and moved about less and less, ultimately lying still. The optic nerve atrophied and developed a characteristic sign, a cherry-red mark on the retina.

Alzheimer concluded the publication with an observation that demonstrated how much he cared about the interests of the disabled:

> The less gifted, the idiots, are predominantly entrusted in Ger-
> many today to nonmedical care. With few exceptions, differences
> of views and an inadequate understanding of the tasks of medical
> research do not foster the cooperation necessary for flourishing
> scientific work.
>
> The little that we know about idiocy we owe to the few idiot
> asylums that are under medical direction and the few clinics for the
> insane that have made accessible a larger collection of material on
> idiocy. However, the great scientific importance of further re-
> search into idiocy well justifies the wish that the clinics turn to the
> study of idiocy more than they have so far and that the asylums for
> the insane and for the idiotic make more of their observation ma-
> terials accessible to scientific assessment.

Alzheimer was an experienced neurologist. He was completely familiar with the method of lumbar puncture (the extraction of cerebrospinal fluid with the aid of a hollow needle from the base of the spine), and he knew
the difficulties in visualizing cells of cerebrospinal fluid to recognize mor-
phologic differences.

For this reason, in 1907 he published "Several Methods of Recording
Cellular Elements of Cerebrospinal Fluid" in the *Zentralblatt für Nervenheilkunde und Psychiatrie*.[29] The plasma cells that he valued so highly could
now be recognized clearly.

Alzheimer was invited to Frankfurt to lecture to the German Association for Psychiatry as an expert on epilepsy. He discussed the congenital
form of epilepsy and said that with his microscope he could see sclerotic
changes and glial growths on the surface of the brain, which appeared in
place of the sunken cortical tissue. Alzheimer enumerated a number of
causes that could be responsible for epilepsy: traumatic brain injury, brain
tumors, certain forms of idiocy, encephalitis, syphilitic diseases, and alcohol and lead poisoning. He emphasized, "Seizures must be prevented at all

costs because the decline of nerve cells runs parallel with the number of convulsive attacks, and a *Krampfschaden* [nerve cell damage from convulsions] emerges."[30]

Alzheimer had thus coined two important concepts: *Krampfschaden* and *Wesensveränderung* (personality change). On the basis of his research on epilepsy, Alzheimer might be regarded as one of the pioneers of a new subject, epileptology, which subsequently established itself at many university clinics. The Center for Psychiatry in Frankfurt still runs an epilepsy outpatient department today, continuing the tradition founded by Heinrich Hoffmann, Sioli, and Alzheimer in Frankfurt.

In 1907 Alzheimer traveled ceaselessly from one congress to the next. Dementia in early and advanced age moved increasingly to the forefront of his work. On May 22, 1907, using his new projection system, he showed microscopic slide preparations of the brain of a 100-year-old man.

Ernst Dupré, an age researcher from Paris, had given him the brain, which Alzheimer dissected in his anatomy laboratory; he then made a brilliant histopathological representation of it. The brain showed neither plaques nor neurofibrillary tangles, that is, abnormal protein deposits and fibers in the nerve tissue, and his audience was comforted to learn that one could reach such an advanced age without falling prey to mental illness.

In Munich Alzheimer had to expand his scientific focus. Kraepelin demanded that he explore not only the exogenous mental disorders—the dementias—but also the psychoses, with an emphasis on dementia praecox (i.e., schizophrenia) and manic depression, or bipolar disorder. Intensive work was carried out in Kraepelin's clinic on the psychiatric theory of illness and the localization of mental illnesses in the brain. Kraepelin also emphasized the binary division of mental illnesses.

Kraepelin had long intended to classify the multitude of psychiatric symptoms according to their origin, their clinical appearance, and their course into categories of illness and to introduce a clinically useful theory of illness. He had pursed this idea as early as his inaugural lecture in 1887, when he became a professor of psychiatry at the Baltic University in Dorpat. Kraepelin's concern was to relate psychopathological phenomena to corresponding histomorphologic changes. Because he thought Alzheimer was capable of developing this classification system, he had brought this promising neuroanatomist first to Heidelberg and later to Munich and bound him to his clinic. Alzheimer fulfilled his expectations. Like Kraepelin, he believed that the pathological anatomy of the central nervous system mirrored psychiatric symptoms: "I do not want to draw any differential diagnostic conclusions from my images but rather just to indicate that they offer an insight into the future histological distinction of different forms of illness among the group of the functional psychoses."[31]

Kraepelin's—and thus also Alzheimer's—theory of disease nevertheless was rebuffed at the annual assembly of the German Association for Psychiatry in Munich in 1906, specifically by Hoche and Boenhoeffer, the so-called anti-Kraepelinians, who regarded any efforts to prove empirically the existence of separate and "natural" categories of illness as vain and rejected the notion that such categories could be distinguished: "There can be no talk of nosological specificity," said Bonhoeffer. Hoche called discussion of this topic fruitless and remarked with slight irritation, "The search for illness types is a hopeless hunt for a phantom!"[32]

Kraepelin was more measured: "What you call a phantom, dear colleague Hoche, is an ideal, one that we cannot perhaps achieve but must nevertheless strive toward."

However, Hoche continued aggressively: "The hope that pathological anatomy will be a powerful aid in the delimitation and division of the represented fields of illness is slight, although this hope has, until now, been the assumption behind all expectations."

Alzheimer, always measured and mediating, replied, "As far as the anatomic doctrine is concerned, I remain, despite Hoche's considerations, a loyal supporter of it. It is not justified to assert that there is no pathological finding at the basis of some mental illnesses as long as we are so far away from a more exact knowledge of the structure of the normal cerebral cortex."

Even Gaupp, former chief physician in Munich, turned against them and took Hoche's side: "No mental symptoms can be explained from anatomic findings."

Finally, Binswanger found a compromise: "Alzheimer's anatomic doctrine, with proof of a pathological-histologic findings, is valid only for psychoses with irreversible cellular damage. I would expressly exclude cases with reparable damage of the nerve cells—that is, the majority of the acute and toxic psychoses."

Alzheimer remained composed and replied, "I have enough cases where I can verify my anatomic doctrine. Twelve days ago, on April 8, a

Frankfurt patient, Auguste D., died. I have had the clinical record and the brain sent to Munich, and I intend to document that in this case there is indeed an anatomic doctrine."

Of course, Kraepelin's doctrine was not the only subject of dispute; the theory of localization was also the object of lively controversy. Karl Kleist, who through exact localization assigned psychiatric peculiarities according to kinds of defined brain damage, was in 1908–09 guest doctor at the Munich clinic and active in Alzheimer's anatomy laboratory.

It was clear to everyone that there were two ways to arrive at new knowledge in psychiatry: One was via nosology, that is, through the examination of the processes of a disease, and the other was through the assignment of symptoms to regions of the brain, the so-called theory of localization.

Alzheimer initially inclined more to nosology than to localization: "We come to a natural summary of the different conditions of illness when we take not localization but rather the variety of diseased tissue processes as the foundation of the delimitation of individual illnesses." The thesis was the content of his most important publication, which asked, "Do we have to presuppose for the various mental illnesses an approximate parallel process of histologic disease?"

In contrast, Kraepelin turned more and more to the principle of localization:

We may hope for further information, especially from the development of an—admittedly interminably difficult—topographic pathological anatomy. The cerebral cortex consists of an initially incalculable number of individual organs, so that the particular local extension of the diseased changes must decisively influence the clinical image.

It is therefore probable that the same disease process can, according to position and extension, produce quite divergent symptoms, as we already know from a series of serious brain afflictions; anatomic research would thus be called on to represent the essential similarity of apparently different forms. On the other hand, the thought arises that anatomically similar processes of disease could of course be substantially distinguished from each other through their particular distribution in the cerebral cortex.[33]

What Kraepelin—at that time the "pope of psychiatry"—formulated quickly became an international standard. He was so convinced about brain localization that at the founding of the German Research Institute for Psychiatry in 1918 (which Alzheimer did not live to see) he instituted a topographic histologic unit directed by Brodmann, who researched the structure of the human cerebral cortex. The success of the unit quickly gained widespread attention.

Another important area of research at the Munich Psychiatric Clinic was the division of the endogenous psychoses into the prognostically favorable, often curable manic–depressive insanity and the unfavorably coursed, incurable dementia praecox, or schizophrenia.

This separation was possible because clearly distinguishable psychiatric categories of illness were present that could be researched using different methods of equal validity in tandem. This was accomplished in Munich under ideal circumstances: Alzheimer was almost always present at Kraepelin's lectures, and he demonstrated there the anatomic characteristics of deceased patients and related them to clinical symptoms. In these demonstrations Alzheimer repeatedly returned to his favorite topic by looking for the corresponding neuroanatomic foundations for a variety of clinical symptoms.

Kraepelin and Alzheimer worked to clearly define clinical pictures throughout their lives because they believed that the nature of an illness could be understood, its causes researched and its outcome predicted, only when the clinical picture was sharply delineated. Gaupp remarked,

> It was no accident that the work brought him together with Kraepelin. Kraepelin's clinical standpoint, and his efforts to consider causes, symptoms, course, and outcome in equal measure in the system of psychoses, were the necessary foundation for Alzheimer's research. The main thing at stake for him was, above all, to uncover different processes of disease, to bring them into parallel with various clinical pictures.[34]

In all the fields of psychiatric research and theory that were pursued at the Munich clinic, Alzheimer was the expert and ideal contact for students and visiting doctors and one of the leading opinion-makers.

On one hand, he had a sober, pragmatic manner, as when he concisely subdivided psychiatry into "organic," or exogenous forms, and "functional," or endogenous forms. On the other hand, he could regularly turn metaphorical, as when he raised the question of whether "psychological degeneration is to be compared to a tree trunk, from which the individual forms of degeneration grow out in diverging branches, or whether there are many separate trunks of degeneration, each with its own roots and own branches."

Alzheimer never gave up the hope that psychiatry would one day achieve what had become a given in other fields of medicine: "the classification of cases of illness according to the illness's cause and its essence with regard to mode of appearance and outcome within particular limits."

However, Alzheimer did not achieve his life's ambition: to distinguish unequivocally the schizophrenias from manic–depressive insanity on the basis of histopathological findings. At the time of his death, his *Histopathology of the Psychoses* remained an unfinished manuscript. Some of his colleagues suggested that the book was almost finished. However, Kraepelin remarked soberly, "After his death only some sketchy beginnings had been worked through to the end; everything else was lost with him."[35]

Proof of Alzheimer's versatility is found in a publication from 1907. He published a detailed article in the *Münchner Medizinischen Wochenschrift* (*Munich Medical Weekly*), "On the Grounds for Termination of Pregnancy in the Mentally Ill."[36]

Paragraph 218 of the penal code was established in 1872; it defined abortion as a crime of killing an unborn person. The grounds for performing an abortion were narrowly bounded at that time. Only an objective endangerment of life through illness during pregnancy justified intervention. A relevant gynecology textbook of the time stated, "Abortion may never be introduced on the basis of subjective complaints alone."

Alzheimer approached the problem with his usual thoroughness and made his remarks extremely vivid through two case histories.

A woman who had already gone through four births without falling ill entered the Psychiatric Clinic in May 1895 because of a depressive condition. In a still deeper depression she is removed from the clinic by her husband against medical advice, soon becomes pregnant, and, at the beginning of September, returns to the clinic in an agitated depression. Great motor agitation, deep anxiety, would like to "cry out loud for inner agitation, fear, and trepidation." Gradually her pathological ideation turns increasingly to her pregnancy. She herself wished for a child, to become healthy. That was a great injustice, because she couldn't feed it; her entire family would have to perish.

Transferred to Eglfing [a psychiatric clinic near Munich], the agitation increases. Persistent refusal of food, constant attempts to harm or kill herself. She had to be held for weeks. Finally a successful, normal birth, and today the mother is at home again, albeit not fully recovered. But here too the depression existed before the birth, and the agitation continued for a good while after it.

Things did not always go as well as described here. Alzheimer also saw the other side of the coin and reported on another case, "knowledge of which I owe to the kindness of Professor von Gudden. A premature birth was induced in a patient suffering from a serious manic agitation. The child died soon after the birth, the mother perished a few days later of puerperal sepsis."

Alzheimer then went over all the essential psychiatric illnesses and stated whether grounds were given for termination of pregnancy. In manic–depressive insanity he saw no grounds for termination; the danger of suicide could be counteracted more effectively and with less intervention through time in a closed ward, he said. He was not convinced of the healing influence of an abortion.

He saw things similarly with regard to dementia praecox. He cited nine case histories in which seven women were already sick when they became pregnant. In no case could birth substantially influence the course of the illness. He saw no grounds for termination of pregnancy in dementia praecox.

Alzheimer did not take an unequivocal position on general paresis because he did not yet know that syphilis was the cause of this disease. However, he did remark that many paretic pregnancies ended with a miscarriage or with a premature birth and that in many cases a living but weak child was born. On the other hand, he emphasized how little most paretics were harmed by birth.

His colleague Binswanger held abortions to be appropriate in special cases of epilepsy. However, Alzheimer noted that it was not unusual to elicit from the case histories of epileptic women that the attacks became less frequent during pregnancy: "That has even passed into an erroneous generalization in popular opinion, and in Munich from time to time epileptic girls or their mothers ask whether it wouldn't be good for the patient to have a child." Alzheimer left inquiries of this kind open but nevertheless held that the influence of pregnancy on the further course of the illness was not harmful.

Regarding hysteria, Alzheimer correctly remarked that pregnancy did not produce hysteria but was undoubtedly an important psychogenic moment that could catalyze hysterical conditions. He relayed an impressive case history to illustrate this:

> A girl from a bourgeois family had been shamefully deceived, feared the disgrace, and, clearly with the serious intention of taking her life, tried to drown herself. Pulled out of the water, she had hysterical seizures. The confession of the motive of her suicide attempt gave her parents cause for the weightiest curses and recriminations. The girl suffered one series of hysterical attacks after the other; in between she showed delirious behavior, spoke of diapers and the gallows, and believed herself to be on straw in prison, quite as if Gretchen in *Faust* had been her model.
>
> Her parents stubbornly refused to bring their daughter to the asylum because that would bring her disgrace into the light of day. It went on for weeks in the same way at home. Then the attacks became less frequent. Meanwhile, the parents had arrived at a calmer view of the situation. From the fifth month of the pregnancy on there was a continuing improvement. The girl later gave birth outside the institution and has remained without hysterical manifestations for at least several years.

In two cases of pregnancy with moderate feeble-mindedness and in three cases of idiocy Alzheimer remarked rather crudely that "no female person can be so stupid in mind and so repulsive in body that she is not exposed to the danger of being sexually abused. The illness is naturally not influenced by the disease, and there is no reason to terminate pregnancy."

In chorea gravidarum (a postinfectious condition characterized by emotional lability, involuntary movement, and hypotonia in pregnancy) and eclampsia Alzheimer saw grounds for termination of pregnancy in severe cases when it could save the mother.

He referred to a case in which, after an induced premature delivery, he saw that the choreatic symptoms did not fade and that blood poisoning occurred during childbirth, which caused the death of the mother; the child died immediately after the delivery. It was generally held that in severe cases of eclampsia it is advisable to induce a premature delivery, and Alzheimer concurred in this publication.

Alzheimer also made a clear statement on the descendants of the mentally ill:

Our research had, until now, primarily turned itself in the direction of degeneration. That there is and must be, however, also a regeneration, a gradual disappearance of pathological dispositions from the genealogical tree, because otherwise humanity probably would already have degenerated completely—this has, so far, been pursued far less.

Perhaps the future will let us see more clearly here and then show other principles to advantage; today we would go on endlessly if we were to see ourselves as justified in placing into the scales the inferior status of the descendants of the mentally ill, and the question of when we have to decide whether a termination of pregnancy is or is not appropriate.

With that Alzheimer distinguished himself very clearly, very early on, from his colleagues Hoche and Rüdin, who later provided the impetus for a terrible development: In 1922 Hoche published his book *Lifting Controls on the Destruction of Lives Unfit to Live: Its Measures and Its Form.*[37]

This concept of "life unfit to live" or "life not worth living" (*lebensunwertes Leben*), as Hoche and his coauthor, Binding, presented it, under the influence of social Darwinism and the heightened economic and cultural crisis after World War I, introduced an intense debate with serious consequences for "euthanasia," the killing of people by doctors out of supposedly humane and progressive motives.

In 1916 Rüdin became director of the genealogical-demographic unit of the German Research Institution for Psychiatry in Munich. As a scientist he distinguished himself primarily with works on the genealogy of schizophrenia. However, he continues to be remembered for writing the medical commentary on the Nazi law on the prevention of congenitally ill offspring, a law he also helped to implement.

In 1909 Rüdin freed Alzheimer from the burden of being Kraepelin's chief physician and deputy. Alzheimer now had time to write a 160-page article, "Contributions to the Knowledge of Pathological Neuroglia and Its Relationship to the Processes of Decomposition in Nerve Tissue," which he published in 1910 as sole author in his house journal, co-edited by Nissl, *Histologische und histopathologische Arbeiten über die Grosshirnrinde* (*Histological and Histopathological Works on the Cerebral Cortex*).[38]

At the end of this very detailed article, which also summarized his previous works, Alzheimer remarked,

We all know that we do not have unchangeable tissue before us in our slide preparations but that we instead have to work with images of equivalence, making constant comparison of how the same methods represent to us normal and pathological tissue parts. Nissl, the real father of the pathological anatomy of the cerebral cortex, has repeatedly emphasized this in many places.

However, we can achieve deeper knowledge in this way, as is proven by the course of development of the pathological anatomy of the rest of the body, which in fact works with the same difficulties.

Alzheimer never gave up:

A feeling of resignation has never stolen upon me. However, my knowledge of the extraordinary difficulties of this field of work has prevented me from ever hoping that the microscope will solve all the riddles of psychiatry in the near future. When I put together everything that the pathological anatomy of the central nervous system has achieved since the last decade of the previous century, I can well say, it is a good piece of work. I do not want to cite the names and works here for fear of forgetting something important.

The physical examination of the brain certainly is expected to bring about a number of forward steps in knowledge, and we therefore all have reason to be happy about this research method. The physicists of the brain may decide for themselves; we who want to help psychiatry progress with the microscope will not let that disturb us in our work. I am sure that we will not need to fear the scales.

In this wide-ranging publication can also be found seven skillfully colored illustrations, almost all of which were drawn by Alzheimer. They are recognized in the field of histopathology as being of the highest artistic quality.

That Alzheimer could also take critical positions on social questions is demonstrated by an article he published in 1911 under the title "Is the Establishment of a Psychiatric Unit in the Reich Health Office Desirable?" in the *Zeitschrift für die Gesamte Neurologie und Psychiatrie (Journal of Complete Neurology and Psychiatry)*.[39] In this article Alzheimer clearly takes a position on the suggestions of Robert Sommer, the *Ordinarius* (full professor) of psychiatry at Giessen.

According to Sommer, such an establishment ought to have included the following fields:

An administrative unit

A clinical unit, which would concentrate on methods and basic research

A unit for forensic psychiatry, which would be concerned partly with the many reports that made their way into the press— many erroneous—about cases of psychiatric certification

A unit for the theory of heredity and for mental hygiene in the broadest sense

Alzheimer engaged critically with his colleague's arguments and made a strong case for a unit for statistics and institutions as well as for a clinical unit. On the other hand, he believed that integrating a unit for forensic psychiatry into the sphere of activity of the Reich Health Office made less sense: "It is also hard to see how in this sphere, which concerns the administration of justice, the Reich Health Office could accomplish beneficial work."

The perfection of psychiatric examination methods could also be achieved without the assistance of the Reich Health Office, Alzheimer claimed, because numerous clinics and other institutions were equipped with sufficient means to work successfully in this domain. Alzheimer also noted that such a large and wide-ranging institute as the Reich Health Office would have to adapt to the tasks that changing times and new insights into the struggle for the health of future generations would bring. For many realms, however, he held that such a lofty ideal made little sense:

> Just as researchers have been sent to foreign lands to discover the causes of diseases, so too can they be delegated to perform studies in clinics and asylums; one can make inquires domestically everywhere where a special amassment of degenerative appearances makes itself noticeable or have studies done overseas on tribes that degenerate and perish in a shocking way. It is precisely here that one would pick up the trace of some of the causes and laws of degeneration with particular ease.

In his conclusion he nevertheless took a strong position in favor of a central office through which systematic analyses could be guaranteed. The work of such an institute, he said, could contribute a wide range of knowledge that would be valuable in preventing mental illness and degeneration and would be an equal successor to the contribution that the Reich Health Office had already made in fighting physical disease.

The idea of a psychiatric unit in the Reich Health Office was discussed much more and contributed to Kraepelin's founding in 1917 of the German Research Institute for Psychiatry, which later became the Max-Planck Institute for Psychiatry in Munich.

## Auguste D.'s Death

Alzheimer had not forgotten his patient Auguste D. after his departure from Frankfurt in 1903. He had occasionally called there and had also inquired in writing about the state of Auguste D.'s health. Upon Alzheimer's departure from Frankfurt Sioli promised to keep him up to date and to document the course of the disease thoroughly.

On April 9, 1906, an intern from the Asylum for the Insane and Epileptic in Frankfurt called Alzheimer to tell him that Auguste D. had died the previous day. Alzheimer requested that Sioli provide him both with the files on Auguste D.'s illness and with her brain, so that he could examine it

FIGURE 5.10 *The Auguste D. file*

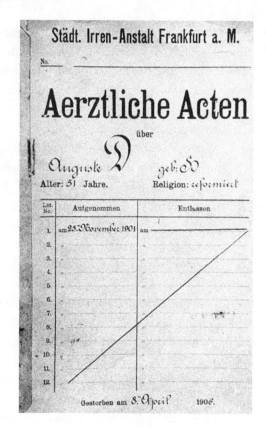

microscopically. Alzheimer believed that behind the clinical symptoms, marked by forgetfulness and jealous fantasies, a new, "peculiar disease," as he put it, could be found in Auguste D.

Alzheimer picked up the Auguste D. file: "Auguste D. remains hostile, screams, and lashes out as soon as one tries to examine her. She also screams spontaneously and then often for hours, so that she has to be held in bed. As far as food is concerned, she no longer keeps to prescribed mealtimes. A boil has formed on her back."

This entry in Auguste D.'s file came from May 1902. The file was carefully assembled, held together with strings on the back. The file cover is deep blue, with nothing written on the back; the cover page is inscribed with the name of the clinic and the most important patient data:

Municipal Mental Asylum, Frankfurt am Main
    Medical files on Auguste D., née H.

*Age*: 51 years
*Religion*: reformed

On an area with numbers running from 1 through to 12 stand the headings "Admitted" and "Discharged." By the number 1 is the date of admission (November 25, 1901); by "Discharged" a horizontal line is drawn neatly with a ruler. The space for entries next to the numbers 2 to 12 is just as precisely crossed out with a diagonal line from the top right to the bottom left corner. On the lower margin of the cover page is printed, "Deceased on April 8, 1906."

On the underside of the front cover page is a card that folds out so that one can find the birth date (May 16, 1850) and name of Auguste D. more quickly.

Alzheimer looked through the file. The clinical history had just arrived with the mail; it contained a total of thirty-one pages, including seventeen pages documenting the disease's history and two on its course. For the most part Alzheimer was familiar with the entries. The original finding came from the admitting doctor, Dr. Nitsche.

In the middle of the files were the four pages Alzheimer had written; the first entry is from November 26, 1901: "What is your name?" The notepaper on which Auguste D. had undertaken her attempts to write, dated by Alzheimer as "26.XI Mrs. Auguste D. Frankfurt/Main," was also still there.

Clinic photographer Rudolph had taken the first photograph, a portrait. Alzheimer's notes ended on November 30, 1901; Dr. Nitsche continued the file after that. The last entry that Alzheimer had made was from June 1902.

At that time Auguste D. was very hostile, screamed, and lashed out when he wanted to examine her. An entry from April 2, 1904, read, "Finding: Completely unchanged."

On November 11, 1904, Auguste D. lay "crouched up in her bed, nestled on the bed coverings etc., senile ergasiomania, continually soiled herself. No longer screams as much as before."

After May 1905 the entries on the clinical record were expanded, with remarks on the course of the illness that several times a month concisely documented the patient's state of health and behavior, with a note on her weight in the right margin. Thus, for example, one reads for June 29, 1905: "Was very loud, came to the bath at 10 o'clock—weight 74 pounds."

On July 12, 1905: "Completely stupefied; always lying in bed with legs drawn up; regularly soiled with feces and urine; never says anything. Mutters to herself, has to be fed. Sometimes becomes agitated without apparent cause, during which time she creates a disturbance through loud screaming and muttering."

On November 7, 1905: "In crouched up posture in bed; mutters to herself quite incomprehensibly, answers questions with a few disconnected words. Plucks with her hands at the bed cover, rummages the bedding into a complete mess, often has to be put in the bath in the evenings because she yells a lot. Takes adequate food, physically recovering somewhat."

December 29, 1905: "Put to bed in the observation room. Lies there rigidly bent up, the knees drawn firmly to the chest. During the attempt to stretch out the legs, strong tension and resistance, screaming very loudly at times, especially nights."

From the clinical record on the course of illness it is clear that she frequently received sedatives. On May 7, 1905, she was not calmed by them, whereas on December 12, 1905, after taking a sedative she slept soundly until morning.

On March 1, 1906, she was again given a sedative because of her tremendous restlessness, did not calm down, and was therefore put in a bath at 11 o'clock. From 1906 until shortly before her death Auguste D. was in the bath every day.

The last fifteen lines of the Auguste D. file describe her last days:

Since the beginning of 1906 a tendency to decubitus ulceration (bedsores); on the sacrum and on the left trochanter [a bone promontory on the left femur] each ulcerated surface about the size of a five-mark piece; very frail, recently a high fever of up to 40 degrees [Celsius]; pneumonia in both lower lobes.

27.–28.3.06: Was constantly very loud; 68 pounds.

29.3.06–30.3.06: Was very loud, into the bath at half past twelve.

6–7.4.06: Was very dazed, wailed from time to time and perspired.

7.4.06: Was dazed throughout the day, temperature at midday 41, in the evening 40 degrees.

8.4.06: Died at quarter to 6.

Auguste D.'s illness thus lasted a little more than four and a half years. As a neuroanatomist, Alzheimer was particularly interested in the autopsy findings:

This morning *exitus letalis*: Death.

*Cause of death*: Septicemia as a consequence of decubitus ulcer; blood poisoning as a consequence of bedsores.

*Anatomic diagnosis*: Mild hydrocephalus externus–internus; water accumulation in the outer and inner cerebral ventricles.

*Atrophie cerebri*: Brain shrinkage.

Arteriosclerosis of the smaller cortical vessels?

*Pneumonia of both lower lobes*: Lung inflammation.

*Nephritis*: Kidney inflammation.

The admission certificate of the Asylum for the Insane and Epileptic, which Sioli had also kindly sent along from Frankfurt, contained details that were new to Alzheimer under "changes":

Mrs. D. is supposed to be moved on April 1, 1904, on the advice of Mr. Karl D., Mörfelder Landstrasse, and per communication of the Social Welfare Office of March 25, 1904.

On August 7, 1902, Auguste was already supposed to have been moved to another clinic because of her husband's difficulties in meeting payments. Alzheimer was able to prevent this because at that time he already knew how important the case of Auguste D. later would be for him. For this reason Mr. D. had been written to at this time, "With reference to the negotiations that took place with you we hereby inform you that the transfer of your mentally ill wife to the Mental Asylum in Weilmuenster will not take place for the time being."

Before this were many visits by the husband, D., who on June 19, 1902, declared to the Social Welfare Office that he paid the full costs of third-class care, 2 marks a day for his wife every month, which he verified by presenting receipts from the payment office. Auguste D. therefore was not indigent and would not be cared for at public expense.

Nevertheless, it was possible that she would have to be transferred. On the same day a letter was very quickly answered in Frankfurt, and the head of the provincial government made a note to the Asylum for the Insane and Epileptic that "with the transfer to an asylum we would necessarily also have to consider the transfer of a larger number of self-paying patients and would next have to review previous applications. We therefore permit ourselves to remain by the present application and leave to our discretion temporarily holding it back until a larger number can be sent in to the head of the provincial government."

Through skilled negotiation and numerous certificates Alzheimer could prevent the transfer of Auguste D., who was so important to him. His efforts were supported by additional certificates personally issued by the director of the asylum: "The above-named D. suffers from a brain disease that has already led to severe stupor and is accompanied by states of intense agitation. The disease offers no hope of recovery."

Sioli sent this letter on January 28 to the First District Attorney at the Royal District Court, in response to a January 21 request for a statement on Auguste D.'s condition. An exchange of letters from 1904 reported that "the costs of care for Mrs. D. will henceforth be collected directly," an arrangement Dr. Sioli confirmed a few days later.

The last letter dates from April 5, 1904: "Auguste D., née H., suffers from a brain disease that has already led to a substantial feeblemindedness and appears with actual states of agitation. The disease offers no prospect of recovery." After that it became clear that Auguste D. would remain in the Asylum for the Insane and the Epileptic in Frankfurt am Main until further notice.

After the file arrived, Alzheimer noted again on an admission form all that he remembered about Auguste D. and what he could glean from the file. On the pink-colored form he entered by hand:

*Name*: Auguste D.

    *Occupation*: Railroad clerk's wife.

    *Heredity*: Mother suffered from seizures after menopause.

    *Prehistory, findings at admission and course*: Always healthy, happily married, only one daughter, no miscarriages. Changed in the last half a year. Jealous fantasies. Decline in memory, frequently during food preparation. Pointless puttering about in the home. Fear of people she knows well. Hid all manner of objects, which she then could not find. Appeared not to know her way about. At admission completely helpless behavior. Completely temporally and spatially disoriented, extraordinarily resistant.

Behaved quite helplessly, poured water on the faces of other patients in the room, says in response to inquiries that she wants to tidy up. Some paraphasic phrases and perseveration in spontaneous speech. Omits letters and syllables when writing. Clearly does not understand some questions directed to her; to others she gives answers that show that she has understood the meaning. Appears to hallucinate.

For a while, as if in a delirium of activity, she carries bedding about and wants to tidy up. Often implies that the doctor intends to do sexual things with her, rules it out indignantly, and throws him out of her house. Screams a great deal in a meaningless way, has intense fear. Repeats paraphasic phrases. Strenuously resists everyone. Lies crouched up in bed in the last year, constantly turns everything away, speaks incomprehensibly. Died after four-year illness in hospital as consequence of decubitus ulcer. Brain atrophy.

This was the kind of form that Kraepelin predominantly used in revising his textbooks to discover and describe new diseases. Alzheimer was aware that these findings, because of the limited space on the form, could represent only the essential in telegram style.

On the other hand, he recognized from the course of the disease and from the initial microscopic examinations of the brain that Auguste D.'s was a remarkable case. He thanked Sioli for letting him have the case history and the spinal cord and brain and also explained to him why he wanted to examine this case in such detail:

It was a peculiar clinical picture . . . in a woman of menopausal age who developed . . . mental disorders without attacks, in which from the very beginning misrecognition of situations played a role and which soon increased to a complete helplessness and to mind blindness [visual agnosia]. At first it did not appear that the corresponding areas in the brain were afflicted, but they soon made noticeable a striking weakness of memory.

Alongside that appeared, often only faintly, focal signs, paraphasic phrases, perseveration, aphasia, and agraphia. The

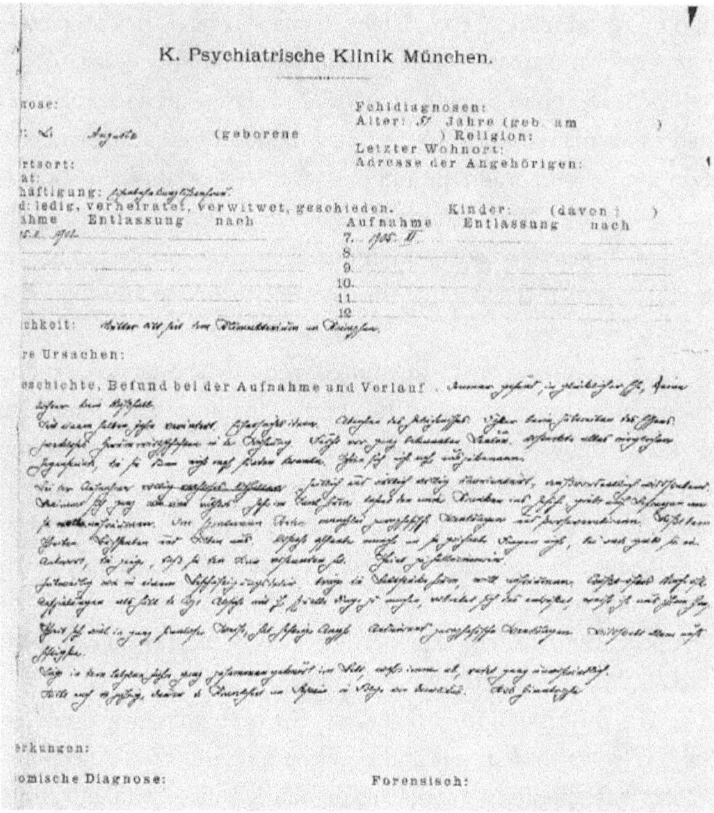
K. Psychiatrische Klinik München.

nose:
Fehldiagnosen:
Alter: 51 Jahre (geb. am )
: Auguste (geborene
) Religion:
Letzter Wohnort:
rtsort:
Adresse der Angehörigen:
at:
häftigung:
d: ledig, verheiratet, verwitwet, geschieden.
Kinder: (davon )
ahme Entlassung nach
Aufnahme Entlassung nach
7.
8.
9.
10.
11.
12.
chkeit:
re Ursachen:
eschichte, Befund bei der Aufnahme und Verlauf
erkungen:
omische Diagnose:
Forensisch:

FIGURE 5.11 *Report on findings about Auguste D., written by Alzheimer in April 1906*

patient died during an increasing stupor after decubitus ulcers had developed. Paralysis and actual manifestations of spasticity did not appear.

In conclusion he advised Sioli of his intention to present the case at the 37th Assembly of the Southwest German Psychiatrists in Tübingen in November 1906.

## *Disappointment in Tübingen*

Only six months remained until November 1906, so Alzheimer set to work with great enthusiasm. The brain was subjected to precise analysis—at first macroscopically and later also microscopically—in the anatomy laboratory by Alzheimer and by Perusini and Bonfiglio, the visiting doctors from Italy.

All three agreed that what they had before them was a peculiar clinical picture. Anatomically it was characterized by an atrophy of the cerebral cortex, with cellular failure on a large scale and a distinct fibrillar disease of the nerve cells, dense growth of fibrous glia, and formation of numerous rodlike glial cells. To their surprise, they found deposits of a particular metabolic product in the form of plaques throughout the cerebral cortex, with signs of growth on the vessels.

The pathological process reminded Alzheimer, Perusini, and Bonfiglio of findings that they knew from senile dementia, which appeared only in the elderly. The striking feature of Auguste D. was that the changes were much more far-reaching than in comparable cases of seventy- to eighty-year-old patients, although at her death Auguste D. was just fifty-six years old. Therefore they were dealing with a presenile disease.

Alzheimer was very well prepared as he proceeded to give his lecture on November 3, 1903, at the afternoon session, which went from quarter to three until 6 o'clock.

Eighty-eight scientists participated in the 37th Assembly of Southwest German Psychiatrists in Tübingen,[40] including Oswald Bumke from Freiburg, who in 1917 wrote an important textbook on mental illnesses. From Bumke comes Bumke's sign, the absence of the pupillary reflex in schizophrenia. Binswanger's disease is named after Otto Binswanger from Konstanz. His nephew Ludwig also became famous for founding *Daseinsanalyse* (existential analysis).

Hans Curschmann, for whom Curschmann–Batten–Steinert syndrome (myotonic dystrophy) is named, was also present. This disease is characterized by weakness and thinning of the muscles (especially in the face and neck), cataracts, hypogonadism, frontal balding, and cardiac abnormalities.

Albert Döderlein of Tübingen, after whom Döderlein's glands are named, sat in the first row; next to him was Robert Gaupp, also from Tübingen, who distinguished himself with works on paranoia, which he studied in the famous case of the mass murderer Wagner.

Alfred Friedrich Hoche, a psychiatrist from Freiburg known as a mocking critic of Freud and of Kraepelin, came from Frankfurt. Carl

Gustav Jung, from the Burghölzli-Spital in Zürich, was also present; he was chief physician under Eugen Bleuler and later developed analytic psychology. Also present was Ludwig Merzbacher from Tübingen, after whom Merzbacher–Pelizaeus disease (a form of leukodystrophy) is named. Of course, Alzheimer was especially happy to see his old friend Nissl from Heidelberg again.

After Bürker from Tübingen finished his talk on the thermodynamics of the muscles, the chair, Hoche, announced the next lecture: "Doctor Alzheimer from Munich will now present 'On a Peculiar, Severe Disease Process of the Cerebral Cortex.' Esteemed colleague Alzheimer, you have the floor."

With his practiced, clear voice Alzheimer reported on the case of Auguste D. and laid out his lecture clearly with brilliant slides.

My former clinical director, Prof. Sioli, kindly gave me the brain and spinal cord to examine.

From a clinical perspective my Auguste D. case already offered such a distinctive clinical picture that it could not be classified among any of the known illnesses. I will describe it to you in what follows.

A woman fifty-one years of age showed jealous fantasies about her husband as a first sign of illness. Soon a rapidly increasing weakness of memory made itself noticeable; she could no longer find her way around her apartment, carried objects here and there and hid them, from time to time she believed that someone wanted to kill her, and she began to cry out loud. In the asylum her behavior bore the stamp of complete helplessness.

She was temporally and spatially completely disoriented. Occasionally she remarked that she didn't understand anything anymore, that she didn't know her way about. Sometimes she greeted the doctor as if he were a visitor and excused herself for not being finished with her work; sometimes she screamed out loud that he wanted to cut her, or she turned him away, full of indignation, with an expression that indicated that she feared an attempt on her womanly honor from him. From time to time she was completely delirious, carried her bedding around with her, called out to her

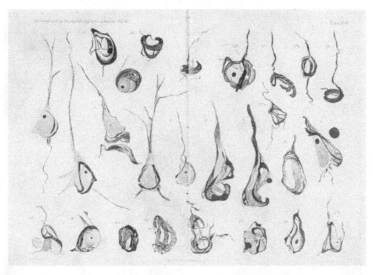

FIGURE 5.12 *Auguste D.'s neurofibrils*

husband and her daughter, and appeared to have auditory hallucinations. She often cried out for hours in a horrible voice.

Every time she was unable to understand a situation, she started to scream loudly when one wanted to examine her. Only through constantly repeated efforts was it finally possible to ascertain a few things.

Her memory was most severely disturbed. If one showed her objects, she generally named them correctly, but immediately afterward she forgot everything again. While reading she skipped between lines, reading each letter individually or with senseless pronunciation. When writing she repeated individual syllables several times, left others out, and fizzled out very quickly. Speaking, she often confabulated and used paraphasic expressions (*milk jug* instead of *cup*). Some questions she obviously did not grasp.

She appeared no longer to know how to use individual objects. Her gait was undisturbed, she used her hands equally well, and the patellar reflex was present. The pupils reacted. Somewhat rigid radial arteries, no enlargement of the heart, no albuminuria.

In the course of her illness, signs that could be interpreted as focal symptoms emerged, sometimes more vividly, sometimes less

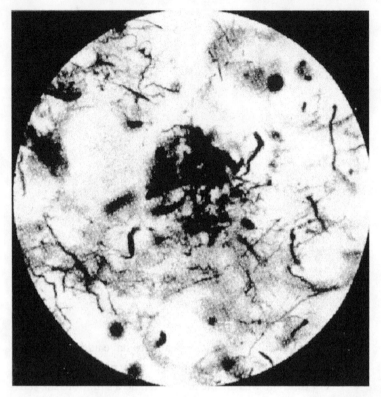

FIGURE 5.13  *Auguste D.'s plaques*

so. In contrast, her general stupor progressed. After four and a half years of illness death intervened. At the end, the patient was completely dull and lay bedridden with her legs drawn up to her, wet the bed, and, despite all care, had contracted decubitus ulcers.

I come now to the details and the slide preparations. The autopsy revealed a regularly atrophied brain without macroscopic lesions. The larger brain vessels had changed arteriosclerotically.

Slide preparations made with the Bielschovsky silver method show remarkable changes in the neurofibrils. In the interior of a cell that otherwise still appears normal, one or a few fibrils stand out through their thickness and impregnability.

The first illustration, please!

Upon further examination, fibrils that run parallel were seen to change in the same way. Then they merge into thick bundles and gradually rise to the surface of the cells. Finally, the nucleus decays, and the cells, and only a crumpled bundle of fibrils indicates the place on which a ganglial cell had lain.

Because these fibrils were stained differently from normal neurofibrils, a chemical conversion of the neurofibrils must have occurred. This may well explain why the fibrils survived the decay of the cells. The conversion of the fibrils appears to go hand in hand with the deposit of a pathological metabolic product in the ganglial cell that remains to be more closely researched.

Second slide!

About one to three quarters of all ganglial cells of the cerebral cortex show such changes. Numerous ganglial cells, especially in the upper cellular layers, have completely disappeared.

The third slide, please! Spread over the entire cortex, especially numerous in the upper layers, one finds millet seed-sized lesions, which are characterized by the deposit of a peculiar substance in the cerebral cortex.

The fourth slide, please!

I want to explain this peculiar substance to you in more detail. It can be recognized even without staining, but it seems to be extremely refractory to staining.

The glia have formed substantial threads, and alongside them, many glial cells show large fatty deposits. An infiltration of the vessels is completely missing. On the other hand, we can see signs of growths on the inner vascular walls and, in places, new vascular formations.

Taken all in all, we clearly have a distinct disease process before us. Such processes have been discovered in great numbers in recent years. This observation suggests to us that we should not be content to locate any clinically unclear cases of illness in one of the familiar categories of disease known to us to save ourselves the effort of understanding them. There are undoubtedly far more mental illnesses than are listed in our textbooks. In many such cases, a later histologic examination will allow us to elucidate the case. But then we will also gradually be able to clinically separate individual illnesses from the big disease groups of our textbooks and clinically define them more sharply. And with that I would like to conclude my remarks.[41]

No one answered to the chair's call for responses. Nor did a further request encourage anybody to pose a question. And even Hoche, the chairman, who normally would have been obliged to rush to the speaker's aid, remained in his place, distant and without comment. Alzheimer was confused because he was accustomed to becoming entangled in lively discussions. Had his colleagues not understood him this time?

The chair remarked, "So then, respected colleague Alzheimer, I thank you for your remarks; clearly there is no desire for discussion," and called on colleagues Frank from Zürich and Bezzola from the Clinic Castle Hardt to present "On the Analysis of Psychotraumatic Symptoms."

Because C. G. Jung, a close collaborator of Sigmund Freud and a champion of his psychoanalytic theory, was there, Freudian psychoanalysis once more was discussed at a psychiatric conference.

In May, at the 31st Assembly of the South German Neurologists and Psychiatrists, Professor Gustav Aschaffenburg from Cologne had passed a withering judgment on Freud in his lecture, "The Relations of Sexual Life to the Emergence of Nervous and Emotional Illnesses."[42]

Then Aschaffenburg prepared to launch his critique: "If masturbation appears in a more favorable light"—he had previously spoken about the reassuring enlightenment of conversation—"then it is undoubtedly false to say, as Freud does, that hysterical symptoms almost never appear as long as the patient masturbates but rather during abstinence."

Aschaffenburg's provocative lecture was published in the *Münchner Medizinische Wochenschrift (Munich Medical Weekly)*, and there it continued, "Through Freud's works the entire sexual life has been shoved into the foreground of the view of the neuroses in a thoroughly garish manner."

He cited Freud himself: "In typical cases of neurasthenia it was regular masturbation or frequent pollution; in the anxiety neuroses it was factors such as coitus interruptus, . . . in which the moment of unsatisfactory discharge of the stored up libido appeared as the common denominator."

Aschaffenburg wrote further, "Freud has now gone so far in his latest work as to demonstrate onanism and sexual perversion in infants." Finally, Aschaffenburg's publication ended, "The doctor has above all the duty not to harm, and it is impossible for this danger to be completely avoided with the Freudian method."

Alzheimer also had discussed psychoanalysis with Kraepelin. In the seventh edition of Kraepelin's textbook, published in 1904, the concept was not yet mentioned; in the next edition psychoanalysis was discussed extensively.

Alzheimer knew his boss's position on psychoanalysis as practiced by Freud and his followers, who, according to Kraepelin, aimed

> to bring to the light of day hidden, repressed ideas, especially memories. The procedure is represented as having the patient lie there calmly and narrate for one to two hours everything that occurs to him, including dreams, to the doctor, who remains unseen throughout.
>
> These confessions—somewhat influenced by the doctor's questions and remarks—are to be continued (in some circumstances for years) until the suspected complex is found. Association experiments with subsequent precise discussion of the connections that may indicate a disorder can also be drawn upon.
>
> It is clear that, on one hand, this extremely intensive procedure is certainly appropriate for giving the doctor a very deep insight into the mental life of the patient. On the other hand, the few extensive reports published so far about this procedure show that an extraordinarily strong and one-sided influencing of the patient takes place via the ideas that the doctor has in mind and, finally, that the attainment of the result sought ultimately demands interpretive skills that obviously only a select few know how to practice. The procedure therefore can never be of general value, at least as long as it has its current goals.

In the presentation that followed Alzheimer's at the Tübingen conference, Frank took a position on Aschaffenburg's criticism of psychoanalysis and remarked,

> It can be explained only by the fact that no one has as yet taken up an in-depth verification of Freud's theories.
>
> That might in part result from the great difficulties of the method, in particular the necessarily large expenditure of time and, not least, from certain prejudices. That these prejudices concern the sexual realm cannot serve as a reason for an unprejudiced researcher to turn away in moral indignation from a method that

allows us insight into the emergence, course, and possibility of curing a range of psychoneuroses that we currently stand before as helpless spectators.

The second speaker, Bezzola, then described a modification of the Freud–Breuer procedure that he called psychosynthesis and concluded that psychoneurotic conditions could best be resolved by reconstructing the causal event or events: "One can give this procedure the name *psychosynthesis* or *traumatosynthesis* to indicate that through a compound of smashed-up fragments under medical supervision a simple, primarily identified experience can be secondarily identified."

After these two lectures a lively discussion was ignited. Hoche, although obliged as chair to assume a certain neutrality, reacted negatively:

> The gentleman lecturers perhaps have the impression that a lack of time has hindered them from a full unfolding of their evidence; I believe that I can say that even had they had complete freedom in this regard they would not have succeeded in convincing the majority of those present. There can be no talk of moral indignation against the Freudian doctrines; on the contrary, it is not anything emotional that repulses most of us about the generalizations of the Freudian "method" but rather very cool and rational considerations; nor would we lack the courage to make more extended experiments if indeed we were more convinced.
>
> Certainly there is much in Freud's theory of the psychoanalysis of hysteria and so forth that is good and new; unfortunately, the good is not new and the new is not good. That a deepened analysis of psychological phenomena and an intensified engagement with the particulars of the individual case can only be of benefit to the medical therapeutic effect, that for the patient a recognition of latent, depressing things and an articulation of them in a place where understanding is present can mean a relief, even a redemption—none of that is new. But all that Freud and others assume about the frequency with which specifically sexual moments are supposed to play a leading role—that is not good.
>
> What, then, have we heard today? That doctors who cultivate psychotherapy with interest and energy have succeeded in sug-

gestively clearing up a series of subjectively agonizing conditions. We have known for a long time that that is possible, and for that one does not need the label of a particular "method" that appears with the pretense of meaning something quite new.

Whoever reads the Freudian "Fragments of an Analysis of a Case of Hysteria" impartially will put it down with a shake of the head; I for my part must confess that it is quite incomprehensible to me how someone could take the trains of thought presented there seriously. I understand it still less when we—those who reject Freud—are reproached that we are not in a position to join the conversation on his theories as long as we have not also applied this "method" ourselves. There just happen to be things for which such a reproach misses the mark because we hold the entire set of premises as fragile; there is therefore a liberatingly comic effect when, as happened in the private discussion, resistance to Freudian ideas is paralleled with the resistance of contemporaries to the Copernican world view.

The entire movement is indeed, for those with a somewhat wider-ranging view, historically understandable; it is a part of a wider current toward the mystical, which is nourished on a surfeit of the anatomic–materialistic way of looking at things. This swing of the pendulum will not last either, and most of us will see the end of these things. In the meantime, we want to protest against it because we do not want to be complicit with something that we see as a fashion and, of course, a bad one, one that, by the way, is full of dangers of all kinds for the medical profession.

At this Jung could no longer remain in his seat:

Freud's theory of hysteria cannot be discarded as nonsense. Sexuality plays a forceful role everywhere. For this reason it is not impossible that many cases of hysteria are reducible to sexual trauma. One cannot assert that Freud is wrong in principle without having applied psychoanalysis oneself. One also cannot declare psychoanalytic method as unfit just like that; that, of course, must first be proven.

Max Isserlin, an intern under Kraepelin, objected,

Verifications in the form of associative experiments following Jung's procedure showed that emotional ideas slow down reaction times, but no data could be found for a standardization of these complexes along the lines of Freudian theory. On the contrary, the emotional character of manifold ideas was demonstrable, as it, indeed, corresponds to the emotivity of the hysterical character. Jung has not been able to find confirmation of his assertion that it is precisely emotive associative disorders that are most easily forgotten—an assertion that has been interpreted from the perspective of the Freudian theory of repression.

After further contributions to discussion, Gaupp attempted to mediate:

I would like to believe that Hoche's stance treats Freud too cursorily. As much as I struggle against the excesses of Freudian theory, I would nonetheless like to warn against discarding the entirety of psychoanalysis as objectionable or worthless. Bleuler and his school [at Burghölzli in Zürich] have, above all, a right to an unbiased testing of the views they have reached through experimentation; a dogmatic condemnation of scientific and practical psychoanalysis appears to me, after the work of Jung and others, impermissible. Great critical caution and a great deal of tact admittedly will be necessary.

The local press reported extensively on the congress and the controversial discussions. The *Tübinger Chronik* (*Tübingen Chronicle*) of November 5 noted the psychiatrists' assembly under the rubric "From City and Country":

On Saturday afternoon at 3 o'clock in the lecture hall of the local Psychiatric Clinic, the proceedings of the 37th Assembly of Southwest German Psychiatrists, for which about ninety participants had arrived, began. First, the previous clinic director, Prof. Wollenberg-Strassburg, greeted the assembly; in mentioning the list of the deceased he regretted in particular the departure this April of Prof. Carl Fürstner in Strassburg. Fürstner, until his passing the president of the assembly, had particularly distinguished himself in neuropathology and was equally important as a researcher, expert witness, teacher, and doctor. He focused in every realm on determining the factual, exact and clear, a real psychiatrist in the best sense of the term. Not only this assembly, but science too, said Wollenberg-Strassburg, had suffered a painful loss in his death. The assembly rose in remembrance of him.

In accordance with the determinations of the chair and the secretary for the assembly, which will cover two days, Saturday and Sunday, a lecture by Prof. Bürker from Tübingen followed, "On the Thermodynamics of the Muscles," in which he addressed the question of how much fuel the muscular system expended.

Dr. Alzheimer from Munich gave an account of a peculiarly severe disease process, which caused a significant shrinkage of the nerve cells within four and a half years.

Seven clinical pictures, some in great detail, were presented by Dr. Frank of Zürich and Dr. Bezzola of Castle Hardt to prove the value of the abreaction of feelings of anxiety by means of hypnotic sleep through the reconstruction of the causal events; according to the doctors, the causes of later melancholic illnesses can be traced back to the experience of feelings of fear in early childhood.

In the theory and, relatedly, the publications of Dr. Freud, the majority of the assembly perceived, as the chair expressed it, an excessively bold intervention into the psyche of the patients entrusted to them; furthermore, the long-term aftereffects of traumata (mental wounds suffered through terror) are, it was said, nothing new, and the general predisposition remains the most important thing. The old Hippocratic view of the derivation of hysteria from sexuality as sole source, according to the majority of the assembly, is mistaken. In conclusion, a speaker from Zürich continued to plead energetically for a fairer evaluation of Dr. Freud, of whom one could not prove that he was wrong.[43]

## On the Tracks of the Mysterious Illness

A year later, in 1907, the page had turned. Although undiscussed and, according to the minutes of the proceedings, "inappropriate for a brief re-

FIGURE 5.14 *Title page of the Allgemeine Zeitschrift für Psychiatrie und Psychisch-Gerichtliche Medizin containing Alzheimer's first publication on Auguste D.*

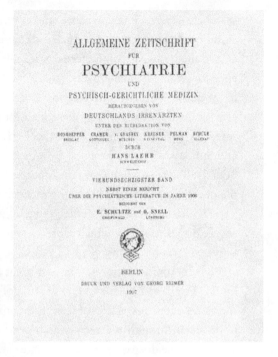

ALLGEMEINE ZEITSCHRIFT
FÜR
PSYCHIATRIE
UND
PSYCHISCH-GERICHTLICHE MEDIZIN

port," Alzheimer's lecture in Tübingen from the previous year appeared in the *Allgemeine Zeitschrift für Psychiatrie und Psychisch-Gerichtliche Medizin* (*General Journal of Psychiatry and Psycho-Forensic Medicine*) under the rubric "Proceedings of Psychiatric Associations" as the second contribution under the title "On a Peculiar Disease of the Cerebral Cortex."

The lecture was printed in full. This publication, hardly noticed in 1907, was cited frequently seventy years later and contributed to the fact that name *Alzheimer's disease* could be traced back to a single medical case, namely that of Auguste D., whom Alzheimer had observed so carefully at the Mental Asylum in Frankfurt.

Alzheimer decided to publish more comprehensively on other patients with presenile dementia. He therefore handed the case of Auguste D. over to his co-worker Gaetano Perusini for further analysis and requested that Perusini look for younger, confused patients among the new admissions at the clinic.

One such patient arrived on March 9, 1907. Mrs. B.A. had lost her memory at age sixty. At the time of admission she was sixty-five. She was euphoric and zombie-like in the clinic, stubbornly and undistractably repeating a few childish-sounding phrases, and exhibited paraphasia. She could not put together a word or phrase from the correct syllables: "Gutele, Memele, Mutele, yes, good, Memele, Mutele, yes so fine, so fine, so finele." Shown objects, she could say only, "Gutele, finele," and she also used terms such as *mustache* instead of *handkerchief* and constantly returned to the same meaningless syllables: "Mutele, Mamele, Mutele, Gutele."

From time to time she made peculiar smacking movements and blew kisses to the doctor. Two weeks later, on March 24, she died. Alzheimer arranged the autopsy and recommended the application of two completely new staining methods in the examination of the brain. Very impressive images were gained with them: "And already under minor magnification the plaques appear with great clarity," noted Perusini.[44]

The district court secretary Sch. L, who also died in 1907, aged more than sixty years old, was examined thoroughly because he too showed early signs of a dementia. On June 20, 1904, he was transferred to the Karthausbruell Mental Asylum, where his behavioral peculiarities worsened. He spoke constantly with his court president and held court sittings by himself, where he usually condemned the accused to death and had one person or another removed from the auditorium. Sometimes he conversed with former lovers, and he declared a fellow patient a whore.

On September 21, 1907, basketmaker R.M., forty-five years old, was admitted. A mental disorder with marked forgetfulness had developed slowly since his fortieth year, and over the years it had developed into a severe memory disorder with complete temporal and spatial disorientation, together with increasing deficiency of intelligence and aphasia.

"For some time he had been unable to hold his urine and peed in the room and in his pants," wrote Perusini, who noted that the patient said things such as, "I can't feed you anymore, the best I can do is to drown myself, so that at least you'll be alone." He could not solve simple equations:

"$2 \times 6$?"

"14."

"$3 \times 6$?"

"That I would have to write down again, there I stand there like an ox!"

To the question, "What is the name of the Kaiser of Germany?" he answered, "The name doesn't occur to me"; when asked the name of the Prince Regent of Bavaria, he answered, "Leopold."

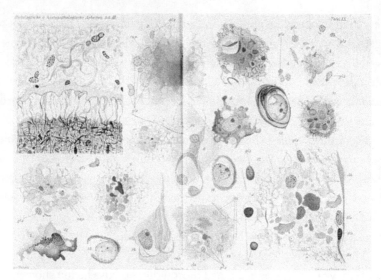

FIGURE 5.15   *Plaque from Auguste D. under number "2" (top center)*

On April 3, 1908, the patient died, and his brain was examined. "Also concerning plaques and the special changes in the neurofibrils and the frequency of their appearance one can only repeat the given description," Perusini and Alzheimer remarked in their comments on this case.

Alzheimer and Perusini thus had four cases on which to publish on after appropriate preparation: the case of railroad clerk's wife Auguste D., fifty-one years old; basketmaker R.M., forty-five years old; Mrs. B.A., sixty-five years old, who lost her memory at age sixty; and finally the sixty-three-year-old district court secretary Sch. L.

The publication, completed in December 1908, appeared in 1909 in the series *Histologische und Histopathologische Arbeiten über die Grosshirnrinde mit besonderer Berücksichtigung der pathologischen Anatomie der Geisteskranken (Histological and Histopathological Works on the Cerebral Cortex with Special Consideration of the Pathological Anatomy of Mental Illnesses)* under the title "On Clinically and Histologically Peculiar Mental Illnesses in Advanced Age," with Perusini as sole author; the editors of the series were Franz Nissl and Alois Alzheimer.

"At the instigation of Dr. Alzheimer I examined the following four cases, all of which are marked by shared clinical and especially pathological anatomic traits," began Perusini. Auguste D. was presented as the first case; for the first time the abbreviation of her surname, *D.*, was cited next to the first name *Auguste*.

The other three cases were described in similar detail and were just as impressively illustrated. In his summary Perusini concluded that in all four cases, "a common main finding can be ascertained, namely a peculiar change in the ganglial cell fibrils and the formation of peculiar plaques, both of which appear in about the same measure and form in all four cases."

Kraepelin was familiar with this publication and its details as well as the personal dialogues with the patients when he started to revise Chapter 8, "Insanity in the Degenerative Age," of his textbook, the previous edition of which had appeared in 1904.

A new edition was urgently needed because of the great demand for the work, as his publisher, Johann Ambrosius Barth in Leipzig, advised him at the beginning of 1907. So Kraepelin began to rework his *Textbook for Students and Doctors* for the eighth edition. The rapid growth of the psychiatric sciences and his many professional duties necessitated that he publish the first volume, on general psychiatry, separately.

Always well informed about his boss's activities, Alzheimer prepared himself at the beginning of 1908 for a long period of deputation, which he assumed from March 11 to April 27, 1908. Kraepelin retreated with his eldest daughter, also a doctor, to Murnau so they could work in peace. Friends had given him use of a house there. He writes of the place in his memoirs:

> We regularly worked here mornings from 8 until 1 o'clock, went for a two-hour walk after lunch, no matter what the weather, mostly in deep snow, rested a little, and then continued work until about 10 o'clock. Apart from her medical studies, my daughter was busy analyzing the results of shooting experiments, which had been carried out at my instigation by the Military Shooting School at Camp Lechfeld. We were interested in determining the influence of moderate doses of alcohol on accuracy, an objective that was achieved faultlessly.

Kraepelin was an outspoken critic of alcohol. In the Munich clinic he issued a strict prohibition on it, although earlier he had extolled it as a sedative for excited patients. Instead, the patients were given a lemonade he had invented, the so-called Kraepelin champagne. In public lectures he supported the establishment of detoxification clinics for alcoholics, an initiative that was successfully opposed by the Ministry of the Interior.

While working on his book, Kraepelin was always up for spontaneous, even far-flung trips, which extended Alzheimer's stint as his deputy:

> One day I unexpectedly received a telegram from America, asking whether I wanted to come to a consultation there. It turned out that I was supposed to travel to Santa Barbara, on the coast of the Pacific Ocean in California. Although my time was very limited because of the urgent work on the book, I decided all the same to take up the invitation. . . . Because I had to severely limit my stay, I was back again after seven and a half weeks and had in this time put on average more than 600 kilometers behind me every day.[45]

Kraepelin's work style was very effective:

> Because I had to process the entirety of psychiatry, it was naturally not possible for me to consult tens of thousands of medical case histories; rather, I had to content myself with the short summaries contained in my notecards. Above all, however, I could not follow up the subsequent fates of all of these patients individually. As a result, great gaps remain throughout; my work no doubt would have been far more fruitful had I filled them in.
>
> Here lie future tasks of great importance. The foolish chatter about the unfruitfulness of clinical psychiatry will soon be silenced when the effort is made to work through really large and carefully documented series of observations.
>
> When I had gained a clear picture of the content of the experience at hand through the indicated path, I then turned to its representation. With the aid of colored pens I highlighted in the extracts from others' works, as well as in the compilation of my own observations, the details that related to the causes, the clinical signs, the course and outcome, the pathological anatomy, and the treatment, and then produced a brief skeleton of all of the material I intended to discuss. The individual sections were built on this skeleton.
>
> Overall, where I could not simply report on others' experiences, I limited myself in the most precise way to the observations

before me, without falling back on general impressions. I can say that every detail of my descriptions of illness is drawn directly from life so that it is influenced only by the natural sources of error of observation and interpretation.

Among this collection of notecards and forms was a description of the case of Auguste D.

Because of Kraepelin's writing, his plans for building his country house, and his many trips ("because I believed I could at this point attend the construction of a country house in Pollenza, I hastily traveled there"), Alzheimer had to stand in for the director of the Munich clinic three more times in 1908: from July 27 to September 16, from October 1 to 20, and from December 23, 1908, to January 6, 1909.

Kraepelin finished punctually: On February 28, 1909, the first volume, *General Psychiatry*, was distributed to bookstores. The second volume, *Clinical Psychiatry*, actually the more important part, first appeared on July 15, 1910.[46]

At this time Alzheimer was constantly needed at the clinic; a corresponding period of deputation appears in his personnel files for March 12, 1909, until April 1, 1909; however, one has to assume that Kraepelin worked uninterruptedly on the second volume throughout 1909 and into the spring of 1910 and that Alzheimer stood in for him at this time, too. Kraepelin thanks him for it in the last paragraph of the foreword of July 15, 1910:

It is with particular satisfaction that I must record here the unfailing support of my long-term, loyal co-worker, Prof. Alzheimer, who enabled me to fit the clinic's usable results in pathological anatomy into my representations in word and image.

But Kraepelin also showed his gratitude to Alzheimer in another way: the expansion of his Chapter 7, "Senile and Presenile Insanity."

In the table of contents, after "Senile Sclerosis of the Brain," the name *Alzheimer's disease* appears. In this section, on page 624, Kraepelin wrote, "Alzheimer described a peculiar group of cases with very severe cellular changes."

The cases named were those of Auguste D., published by Alzheimer in

1907 and again by Perusini in 1909; three further cases of Perusini's, and the individual cases of Bonfiglio and Sartechi.

In writing the text Kraepelin also remembered the patient Johann F., who at fifty-nine years of age also was diagnosed with presenile dementia. Kraepelin saw him for the last time during his extensive rounds on May 31, 1910; at that time he showed a marked ergasiomania.

He was not doing well. He had been a patient of the psychiatric clinic since November 12, 1907. Approximately six months before admission he had become forgetful, could not find his way around, could no longer perform simple tasks or could do so only awkwardly, and just stood around, no longer worried about eating but then eating greedily what was placed before him. He could no longer buy things and did not wash himself; he was presented for admission by the city's charity organization.

As with Auguste D. and many other patients, Alzheimer thoroughly examined Johann F. On September 20, 1907, he approached his bed and asked him,

"What color is blood?"

"Red."

"Snow?"

"White."

"Milk?"

"Good."

"Soot?"

No answer.

Johann F. counted correctly to ten, correctly named the days of the week and the months, and recited the first half of the Lord's Prayer but then could not continue.

"2 × 2?"

"4."

"2 × 3?"

"6."

"6 × 6?"

"6."

He correctly read the clock. He buttoned a jacket properly. He put a cigar in his mouth, struck a match, lit the cigar, and smoked, all correctly. He held coins and checked them on all sides: "That is, that is, there we have, there, there."

Alzheimer asked further, "How many legs does a calf have?"

"Four."

"A person?"

"Two."

"Where does a fish live?"

"In the forest, in the trees?"

Alzheimer, shaking his head, "In the forest, in the trees?"

When on October 8, 1907, Johann F. was asked to write, he picked up a matchbox and tried to write with that.

On June 12 he walked in the garden in a continuous, circular path, maintaining a rapid tempo as long as nobody stopped him, although he was completely bathed in sweat. During this walk he constantly wound the long skirts of his coat around his hand and frantically held them together. In bed he did the same thing with the bed covers. When poked with a needle or tickled on the soles of his feet, he did not react for a long time, and then lashed out at the doctor, to whom he hardly spoke a word. On October 3, 1910, day laborer Johann F. died of pneumonia at age fifty-nine.

Because this patient, undoubtedly with presenile dementia, died after publication of the textbook, Kraepelin could only evaluate the case clinically; in 1911, however, Alzheimer produced an extensive publication on it.[47]

From Kraepelin's extensive experience and his clinical practice finally emerged the definitive text, one that first named one of the most important and well-known diseases in the history of medicine.

Kraepelin masterfully described the symptoms of presenile dementia:

Alzheimer described a peculiar group of cases with very severe cellular changes. They concerned the slow development of an unusually severe mental infirmity, with weak signs of an organic brain disease.

Over the years the patients gradually regress mentally, become weak in memory, impoverished in thought, confused, and unclear. They can no longer find their way around, fail to recognize people, and give their things away. Later a certain restlessness develops; the patients chatter a lot, mutter to themselves, sing and laugh, run about, fiddle around, rub, pluck, and become unclean. Indications of aphasic and apraxic disorders are common; the patients do not understand any requests or gestures, do not recognize objects and images, do not complete any ordered tasks, do not imitate, and do not make any movements to defend themselves against threats, although they find pricking with a needle very uncomfortable.

The speech disorders, above all, are most profound. The patients can produce comprehensible individual words or sentences well but usually fall into a meaningless babbling, in which . . . the frequent, rhythmic repetition of the same toneless syllables stands out; apparently this has to do with a particular form of "fixation." The following transcription may give an idea of this disorder:

"Not good, good, drink myself, not sweet, sweet. The lumpa, have lumpa, have all they all all zam zambrought, sling hen hen all water. She said should slide slide also have there not nope come your houndings not please my mother mother children children God the Lordy now also have of course not made not not hearts heart heart newnew year year. . . ."

Here at least most of the words—and here and there even certain connections—are still recognizable. Later, however, this babbling dissolves into a completely incomprehensible sequence of slurred syllables. During one, admittedly only very incompletely successful attempt to write down something of these expressions, I received the following fragments, produced in rapid, rhythmical sequence:

"Un a so saes sa sa sa sa schosche schosche schosche da da da awae olse ru dis so so so so ro have one o rae sae sae sae sae so sa sa sa sa so it goes taet so so schae you ta teu schae schae schae a ra wa ra se schae schae schae schae."

Finally the patients fall into complete silence, emitting, only when excited, single comprehensible words or meaningless groups of syllables. Writing is impossible. At the same time, the highest conceivable degree of stupor develops. The patients perhaps look up when one turns to them, occasionally smile, but no longer understand a word or a facial expression, no longer know their next of kin, and answer only to direct physical intervention with gestures of irritation and hastily pronounced, ill-defined syllables, in which they might mix a comprehensible curse word here and there.

They are incapable of eating by themselves or otherwise looking after themselves, put into their mouths anything that is put into their hands, and suckle on objects held up to them. From time to time they are restless and probably also frightened.

Physically, one observes more or less strong tensions, predominantly in the legs, general weakness, tripping, uncertain gait, but as a rule no focalized symptoms apart from the aphasic, apraxic, and paraphasic disorders. Many of my patients had occasional epileptiform attacks. The pupillary reaction is perhaps somewhat reduced, as is the skin sensitivity, insofar as that can be tested in cases of stupor; from time to time signs of arteriosclerosis appear.

The final condition represented here can continue with a very gradual worsening or remain seemingly unchanged for many years. Death ensues in the cases I have observed through comorbid illnesses. According to Alzheimer's account, autopsy shows changes that to an extent represent the most severe forms of senile sclerosis.

The drusen [abnormal albumen deposits] were unusually numerous, and almost a third of all cortical nerve cells appeared to have died. In their place lay remarkable crumpled-up, vividly colored fibrillary bundles, obviously as the last remnant of the destroyed cell bodies. The glia showed widespread growth, especially strongly around the drusen. On the vessels signs of light growth could be found only rarely, whereas there were predominant signs of degenerative processes.

The clinical interpretation of Alzheimer's disease is unclear at the moment. Whereas the anatomic findings suggest that we are dealing with a severe form of senile dementia, the fact that the disease from time to time begins at the end of the patient's forties speaks against it. In such cases at least one would therefore have to assume a presenile dementia, if we are not in fact dealing with a peculiar disease process that is largely independent of age.

The clinical picture, with unusually severe stupor, far-reaching speech disorders, signs of spasticity, and seizures, differs clearly from presbyophrenia (a form of senile dementia characterized by defective memory, garrulousness, and confabulations with a cheerful, lively temperament) because it otherwise tends to accompany pure senile cortex changes. There may be relations to one of the earlier pictures presented under the presenile diseases.[48]

As precise as the description already was at that time, there were usually only a limited range of options for treating senile dementia—and thus presenile dementia as well. Thus it seemed that all one could provide was "careful physical care and supervision of the often infirm and frail patient, with regulation of the entire way of life, especially nutrition and digestion, controlling fear with small doses of opium, sleeplessness with baths, careful wrappings, occasional prescription of paraldehyde and veronal. In delirious states of excitement the use of upholstered beds or duration baths, as well as special food (with or without the supplement of a calmative) is more frequently necessary. On the other hand, in the calmer forms of imbecility institutional treatment is in many cases unnecessary and should be replaced completely with care within the family or in a church-run institution," remarked Kraepelin at the end of his chapter.

The well-known hypnotic and sedative veronal (barbital) was put on the market in 1909. Auguste D. did not live long enough to use it, but Kraepelin immediately recognized the medication's value, especially for extremely unruly patients. Veronal was produced by the Merck firm in Darmstadt. Apparently Fischer and Mehring, who developed the drug, gave their sedative the name *veronal* on a conference trip to Verona. Luminal, a well-known phenobarbital preparation, was developed in 1912.

The medical files on Auguste D. that underlay the exploration of Alzheimer's disease were rediscovered in 1995. As the *Frankfurter Rundschau* of June 4, 1997, reported, "For two years Maurer, Volk, and Gerbaldo had searched systematically but in vain in the Institute for City History, in the Hessian State Archive, as well as in the archive of the psychiatric unit of the University Clinic for files of patients who matched the known initials. They brought twelve 'A.D.' cases to light. None fit with Alzheimer's account. Accident helped out: The historical file had been stored in the cellar of the clinic under a completely incorrect year—with the documents of patients after 1920—and that is where the doctors stumbled across the file in December 1995 during yet one more effort to find it."[49]

## Farewell to Munich

In autumn 1906 Alzheimer became Kraepelin's leading chief physician after his predecessor, Robert Gaupp, was called to Tübingen.

Kraepelin had promised Alzheimer that he could step down after an appropriate period: "I would make an effort in the next few years to find someone who could take over his position." However, the "appropriate period" lasted three years. By February 22, 1909, Alzheimer finally lost his patience. In a written application he requested release from his position as chief physician on the grounds that he needed all his time for scientific research.

He further increased the pressure on his boss by petitioning for leave during the summer semester on March 1, 1909, to be able to finish his "Studies on the Motor Foundations of Mental Disorders and Histological Changes in Epilepsy." He said that he had to perform examinations in large epileptic asylums because the patients in a psychiatric clinic such as Munich's were housed for only a short time. Because this plan conflicted with his teaching duties, he requested an exemption for the summer semester. Kraepelin approved the petition and forwarded it to the senate.

Only Ernst Rüdin was considered a fitting successor; he was ten years younger than Alzheimer and had been a student of Kraepelin in Heidelberg. In his letter to the State Ministry Kraepelin wrote that "Alzheimer [should] continue his work as a scientific assistant and Dr. Ernst Rüdin [should] become his successor."[50]

On March 20, 1909, both applications were approved by Prince Regent Luitpold himself, whereby it was also noted that Dr. Rüdin could begin the position at an annual salary of 3000 marks.

Alzheimer had not long been free of the office of chief physician and working as a scientific assistant when on December 30, 1909—five years after his *Habilitation*—he learned that Prince Luitpold had awarded him the title and rank of extraordinary professor for the duration of his term as privatdozent.

Therefore, after April 1909 Alzheimer could work more on science, which initially led him to take over editorial duties for a specialized psychiatric journal that Kraepelin had been planning.

Kraepelin did not need any great powers of persuasion: "Alzheimer did not know how to coolly turn down urgent requests when he believed them to be justified. When in 1909 the plan for a new psychiatric journal surfaced and I had to ask him whether he would be prepared to take over leadership of it, I was surprised by his immediate acceptance."[51]

Thus in 1910 an important specialist journal emerged, the *Zeitschrift für die Gesamte Neurologie und Psychiatrie* (*Journal of Complete Neurology and Psychiatry*), for which a neurologist and a psychiatrist shared editorship. Berlin neurologist Max Lewandowsky was responsible for the neurologic part, Alzheimer for the psychiatric. Managing this journal took a substantial part of Alzheimer's work time, and he remained the editor until his death in 1915. Thirty volumes appeared during those years.

Alzheimer reserved for himself the first publication in the very first volume and wrote a nineteen-page article, "Diagnostic Difficulties in Psychiatry," which he finished on February 15, 1910.[52] Alzheimer's hard work can be seen in the fact that the first volume contains both his contribution on diagnostic difficulties and another article, "Degeneration and Regeneration of the Peripheral Nerve Fiber."[53]

At last, with his assumption of the editorship of the journal, in 1910 Alzheimer became a candidate for a chair in psychiatry. The name *Alzheimer's disease* had become known worldwide among specialists, and word had spread that Alzheimer was not only an important researcher but also a good clinician with extraordinary speaking abilities.

> Thus in many ways the special note of this mental degeneration already resonates throughout the entire life of manic-depressives, hidden only by social structures and the possibilities of social activity, but then at a certain time it rings out, drowning out everything else: the tendency to develop abnormal moods from inside out, now with elevated mood, fleeting trains of thought, and the need for activity; now with depression, impediments or inhibitions in the development of thoughts and, as we now also know, sometimes appearing with a mixture of both.[54]

Alzheimer's activity in Munich from 1903 until 1912 was his most fruitful creative period, and Nissl describes it thus:

> Purely matter-of-fact in his representations, averse to every exaggeration and to speculative fantasies, free of a personal rancor in disputing other points of view, and filled with a glowing enthusi-

asm for that which he fought for, he was not only a defender but also a recruiter for this direction in research.[55]

At the same time, Alzheimer was wholeheartedly a psychiatrist. Whether in Frankfurt, Heidelberg, or Munich, in these years Alzheimer always worked intensively as a clinician; his drive to do research, to diagnose, and to heal sprang from this source.

Then in 1912 he was offered the position of full professor of psychiatry at the Psychiatric Clinic of the Silesian Friedrich-Wilhelm University in Breslau. Gaupp, his former colleague, who had already occupied the chair of psychiatry at the University of Tübingen since 1906, congratulated him: "When he was appointed to Breslau all of his friends were very happy for him because they knew how much he was drawn by the important duties that he had to perform there."[56]

A dear wish of Alzheimer's was also fulfilled, and despite his great modesty, he was very proud. Kraepelin pinpointed it precisely, remarking that he thought he noticed in Alzheimer a discontent that for so long his formal position had not been commensurate with his intellectual importance and that it made him proud when he finally found well-deserved recognition through the appointment in Breslau.

However, Alzheimer's friend Franz Nissl appeared to feel otherwise: He later relinquished his own chair in clinical psychiatry to return to Munich and to take over the direction of the histopathological unit.

Alzheimer did not hesitate to accept the position. On July 30, 1912, he wrote to the dean of the Munich faculty:

After I, through a resolution of his Majesty the Kaiser and King of Prussia of July 16, 1912, was named to the position of full professor of psychiatry and neurology and director of the Psychiatric Clinic at the University of Breslau, I most respectfully present to the dean of the High Medical Faculty of the University of Munich the request to apply to the Royal Ministry to release me of my function as privatdozent of the medical faculty.[57]

His petition was forwarded to the academic senate on July 31, 1912, and Prince Regent Luitpold approved it shortly thereafter. Kraepelin nevertheless let Alzheimer leave only reluctantly and commented, "When Alzheimer in 1912 received the appointment to Breslau, he accepted it, although I had the feeling that the best that he had to offer our science would thereby be lost. The new, stressful, and hectic activities that awaited Alzheimer appeared, nevertheless, to satisfy him."[58]

The appointment to the chair of psychiatry at Breslau had not fallen into Alzheimer's lap. In March 1912 the members of the appointment commission in Breslau compiled a ranked list of candidates to succeed Prof. Karl Bonhoeffer, who had been appointed to the Charité in Berlin. They had a choice of four reputable candidates.[59]

In first place was the full professor of psychiatry at the University of Zürich, Dr. Eugen Bleuler, a researcher of outstanding originality with a stimulating direction in research. He was active in brain anatomy and brain pathology and had written a work on schizophrenia, among other things. As director of a large institution, he had already made a substantial contribution in Switzerland. The commission nevertheless conceded that "a certain one-sidedness, partly stemming from the character of his subject matter, attaches to his scientific direction." Yet the faculty was convinced that this one-sidedness could be corrected through the more extensive materials available to him in Breslau.

Alzheimer was nominated to second place and presented as follows: "As a histopathologist of the brain he is a recognized authority of the first rank and has worked with great success on the organic psychoses, general paresis, brain lues, arteriosclerosis, and epilepsy. The value of his histopathological works lies not least in the fact that Alzheimer consistently places the relationship to the clinic and the clinical relationship in the foreground. His works on mental illnesses occurring with arteriosclerosis, brain lues, and stationary paresis can also be regarded as exemplary from a clinical perspective. . . . He is a very good and beloved teacher and a competent and conscientious doctor. The faculty is convinced that he would fill the local position in the best manner."

In third place, equally ranked, stood the chief physician of the Psychiatric Clinic in Breslau, Prof. Paul Schröder, and Prof. Oswald Bumke, chief physician of the Psychiatric Clinic in Freiburg.

These suggestions were sent to the Ministry of Education and the Arts in Berlin. Prof. Friedrich von Müller, director of the internal medicine clinic in Munich, undertook a thorough investigation and, by asking assistants, several older students, and many doctors from Munich, discovered the following:

> My sources, who have attended Alzheimer's clinical lectures, all agreed that Alzheimer was an outstanding teacher of clinical psychiatry. One of my current assistants, who was previously an assistant at the Wollenberg Psychiatric Clinic, currently attends Alzheimer's lectures on cerebral anatomy and is frankly enthusiastic about Alzheimer's teaching.
>
> As I have already been able to convey to you, Alzheimer has already been called in as a psychiatric consultant by doctors from both medical clinics for years and still is today, whenever psychiatric patients show up in our units. My assistants have confirmed to me that Alzheimer knows excellently both how to deal with the mentally ill and how to clarify diagnoses. I myself have repeatedly heard Alzheimer lecture and especially remember two outstanding lectures on hysteria and the differential diagnosis of arteriosclerosis of the brain.
>
> As a person and a character Alzheimer enjoys widespread and deep respect here in Munich. I am firmly convinced that he would be an excellent clinician, and for years we here in Munich have already asked ourselves with regret and wonder why Alzheimer has always been passed over until now."[60]

Alzheimer telegraphed the Ministry of Education and the Arts on June 15, 1912, to indicate that he was inclined to accept the offer at the Breslau clinic. On June 19, Alzheimer came to the following agreement with the Minister for Spiritual and Teaching Affairs:

1. Alzheimer declared himself prepared to assume the full professorship in the Medical Faculty of the Silesian Friedrich-Wilhelm University at Breslau on August 15, 1912.
2. He obliged himself as director of the psychiatric clinic to represent the entire range of mental and nervous diseases in his clinical and theoretical lectures.
3. Alzheimer was informed that he was entitled to a salary of 4200 marks as well as free accommodation provided by the univer-

FIGURE 5.16 *Certificate of Appointment for Alois Alzheimer, signed by Kaiser Wilhelm II*

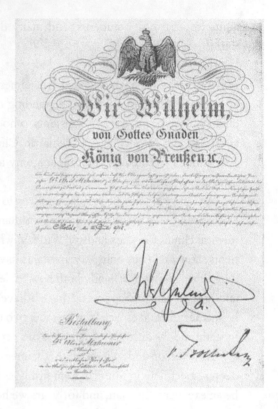

sity, and that the compensation system of bonuses for years of service would not be applied in his case.

4. He was entitled to the honoraria for his lectures of all kinds at the following rates: up to 3000 marks in full, from 3000 to 4000 marks at 75 percent, and 50 percent for higher sums.

5. For the costs of the accelerated move from Munich to Breslau Alzheimer was to receive 1500 marks, immediately payable upon his arrival in Breslau.

Apart from these favorable conditions Alzheimer signed a declaration with which he committed himself

1. In case of an appointment to another institution of higher learning or another kind of position not to enter into negotiations without prior notification of the Ministry of Education and the Arts

2. To begin an appointment only on October 1 or April 1 and only after a period of three months' notice in advance and

3. In the case of resignation within the first three years to repay the moving expenses (1500 marks) after departure from Breslau to the university bursar.

On July 16, 1912, Kaiser Wilhelm II personally signed the certificate of appointment:

We Wilhelm,
> By grace of God
> King of Prussia,
> Announce and hereby decree it to be known that We have magnanimously decided to name Prof. Dr. Alois Alzheimer, previously extraordinary professor at Munich, to the chair of the medical faculty of the University of Breslau. This has happened in the trust that he will remain devoted to Us and Our Royal House in steadfast loyalty and fulfill the duties of the office transferred to him in its full extent with constantly spirited enthusiasm and, in particular, every half year will without fee read a lecture on a branch of the sciences that he is to teach, as well as offer at least one private lecture in his field every semester, against which he should enjoy our highest protection of the rights incumbent upon his current office. We have ourselves Most Graciously certified this appointment and had it stamped with Our royal insignia.

Shortly before Alzheimer took up his position as full professor in Breslau a shadow fell on his joyful mood. The disease Alzheimer had investigated most thoroughly, general paresis, afflicted his long-term laboratory assistant Karl G.

Shaken, Alzheimer received the report by the administrative committee of Munich University and the Ducal Georgian Parish House that the director had sent to the Royal State Ministry of the Interior for Church and School Matters.

The report concerned the transfer into retirement of Karl G. on the grounds that since February 29, 1912, he had been under the treatment of the psychiatric clinic for mental illness. Alzheimer had examined hundreds of cases, made histologic slide preparations, and produced pictures with the camera lucida with him. Now he was asked to authorize "that the ill laboratory assistant G. continue after the thirtieth of the eighth month of this year to be paid his wage temporarily." Alzheimer immediately complied with the request and signed without hesitation.

## 6. Breslau

Kaiser Wilhelm made the following comments in his speech at the 1911 centenary celebration for the Silesian University in Breslau:

> In the old *Piastenstadt* [the Kaiser thereby reminded his audience of the city's Polish past], where the sun of Christianity first shined for the Slavic peoples and the boundary posts of German culture were moved eastward, in the towering German crown of Kaiser Karl IV, which competed in gleam and civil pride with golden Prague, in the old capital city of Breslau, in the capital city of the beautiful land of Silesia, the new university became, according to the will of my ancestors, who now rest with God, a focus of flourishing spiritual life and increasing scientific culture.
>
> Three universities owe their existence to the generous resolution of King Friedrich Wilhelm III; two of them, Berlin and Bonn, bear his name. So that the memory of their founder will also remain alive for later generations at Breslau University, I want hereby to confer his name here too. Thus should my royal thanks and best wishes accompany the Silesian Friedrich-Wilhelm University into its second century. Under this honorable name it will remain what it was, to its own honor, for the fame of the fatherland, and for the progress of mankind.[1]

This university was Alzheimer's destination when in August 1912 he embarked, with not quite all of the family, on his trip. Both Gertrud, seventeen years old, and eleven-year-old Maria were there, as was forty-year-old Maja, without whom the family could no longer be imagined.

Alzheimer's son, Hans, sixteen years old, did not accompany his family to Breslau because he was attending the boarding school in Cloister Ettal, a humanities *Gymnasium* close to Garmisch-Partenkirchen. His father knew that he would be in good hands there because Alzheimer's brother,

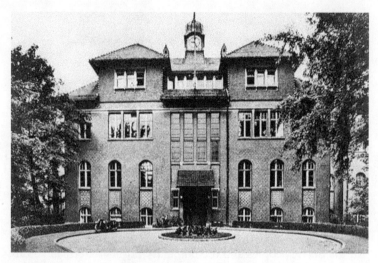

FIGURE 6.1  *The Royal Psychiatric and Nerve Clinic in Breslau*

Karl, was still in Munich, and Hans had an especially close relationship with him; also, he knew that Hans was very happy at school.

On the day of departure, a warm summer day, Alzheimer was exhausted. The efforts of the last weeks, with the disbanding of the laboratory, the illness of his laboratory assistant, the many leave-takings, and the closing down of the apartment—all fatigued him. Without knowing it, he must have already been acutely ill during the journey. Kraepelin later spoke of an "infectious angina with nephritis and inflammation of the joints, which he took with him on the trip to his new place of residence. He was never able to recover from it."[2]

Other colleagues also reported that Alzheimer was already ill on the train, and immediately after his arrival in Breslau had to go to a sanatorium. From then on he experienced shortness of breath and cardiac palpitations at the slightest exertion.

This was a situation that Alzheimer, a man who otherwise radiated strength, a giant of a man with a fighting spirit and extreme sensitivity, could not accept. Nevertheless, these symptoms marked his few years in Breslau and limited the expression of his abilities. At first, Alzheimer would not be deterred; still mentally active and optimistic despite his illness, he set to work.

Alzheimer knew the city only from the visits he made in June 1912 when he was carrying out appointment negotiations. Breslau, the capital city of the Prussian province Lower Silesia, which lies on the River Oder, was at this time the seventh largest city in Germany and counted half a million inhabitants, including 300,000 Protestants, 180,000 Catholics, and about 20,000 Jews. Many impressive churches and high towers rose above the horizon, and above it all the Elisabeth Church tower stood like a giant; because of the fifteen bridges that spanned the width of the Oder, Breslau was also called the Venice of the East.

The Silesian Friedrich-Wilhelm University, with about 4000 students, was the capstone of the educational system; the university library contained more than a half a million volumes. Breslau also home to an agricultural college, the Music Conservatory, and the Academy for Fine Arts and Arts and Crafts.

For the Alzheimers Breslau was particularly attractive, equipped with nine museums and five theaters, although at first sight the possibilities for excursions did not appear to be as splendid as those in Munich. Still, Alzheimer promised his daughters excursions into the Katzen and Riesen mountains and steamer trips through the Oder woods.

His workplace and its furnishings satisfied him in every respect. Alzheimer's appointment included the use of a stately home that stood on the grounds of the clinic, to which the clinic director had always been entitled.

The house, still numbered Auenstrasse 42, stands in the southwest section of the grounds of the psychiatric clinic and was in Alzheimer's time a part of the outpatient clinic. The house, made of brick with half-timbered embellishments in the top floor, has been preserved to the present day, although there have been several changes inside, and today it houses a kindergarten and a health and counseling center. The area around the Oder was popularly known as the *Katastrophenecke* (catastrophe corner) because the fire station, registry office, Royal Psychiatric Clinic, and St. Laurentius Cemetery are clustered there.

An advertisement for the Royal Psychiatric Clinic in the *Breslauer Zeitung* (*Breslau Newspaper*) informs us about Alzheimer's activities at the university:

Consultation hours in the outpatient clinic weekdays from 9 to 11 o'clock in the morning
   Administrative hours weekdays from 8 to 1 o'clock and 3 to 6 o'clock

Director: Dr. Alzheimer, professor

Eighty beds. Admissions daily during the week, but decisions about admission will be made only after an examination by one of our doctors has taken place.

The costs of treatment and board come, in first class, to 8 marks a day for citizens, 9 marks for foreigners; in second class 5 and 6 marks per day, respectively; and in third class 2 and 3 marks, respectively; members of professional associations pay 2.50 marks per day in third class; in the first and second classes they also retain the right to claim a professional honorarium.

Alzheimer announced his private outpatient clinic and was listed in a register of specialist doctors: "For nervous and mental illnesses. Alzheimer, Alois, Auenstr. 42, T. 4335. Daily, except Wednesdays, afternoons 4 and 5 o'clock and also Saturdays."[3]

The clinic was part of an outstanding tradition; before Alzheimer, such well-known directors and scientists as Neumann, Wernicke, and Bonhoeffer had worked there. It is with good reason that this tradition has been called the Breslau school of psychiatry.

Heinrich Neumann, the first director, was one of the earliest representatives of the profession and is considered one of the founders of the unified psychosis concept. According to this view, there are no clearly separable units of illness; rather, the different manifestations of insanity are considered successive stages that represent the changing expression of the same fundamental psychotic disorder.

The second director, who worked from 1885 until 1904, was Carl Wernicke. Wernicke's speech center and Wernicke's aphasia (sensory aphasia), an inability to understand speech despite the ability to speak fluently, are named after him. In 1881 a clinical condition was named after him: Wernicke's encephalopathy or Wernicke's syndrome, a brain disorder that appears primarily in conjunction with severe alcoholism. From him also came such concepts as anxiety psychosis, hallucinosis, motor psychosis, and presbyophrenia.

The third director, from 1904 to 1912, was Karl Bonhoeffer, from whom the principle of exogenous reaction types comes. According to this principle, all causes of illness from outside the brain, such as infections and poisonings, produce the same symptoms. The Breslau Clinic was built under his direction in 1906–1907 at a cost of 1 million marks. It lies about 700 meters north of the complex of university clinics and was divided into two main buildings, each of which contained three units. A total of 700–900 patients per year were admitted according to the type and severity of their illness. About 2000 patients were treated in the outpatient clinic.

Bonhoeffer wrote in his memoirs about the last five years of his service in Breslau: "The five years after the opening of the clinic, the years 1907 until 1912, passed in satisfying clinical scientific work, predominantly in the field of the symptomatic psychoses and psychogenic mental reactions." In 1912 Bonhoeffer left to take a position in Berlin, and Alzheimer became his successor.

The name *Alois Alzheimer* surfaces in the lecture directory of the University of Breslau for the 1913 summer semester. Instruction included lectures on the subject of psychiatry with patient presentations, exercises in anatomy and the pathology of the cerebrum, and lectures on the histology and histopathology of the nervous system. Alzheimer held all lectures and exercises at precisely the same times of day.

In addition to directing the clinic and teaching, his duties included work in the pathology institute, further consultations (twice a week), and discussions of cases in pathological anatomy and histology, which took place Tuesdays and Fridays from 7 to 8 A.M. and Saturdays from 7 to 9 A.M..

Alzheimer was also director of training in histopathology; the courses took place Tuesdays from 3 to 5 P.M., Thursdays from 3 to 4 P.M., and Saturdays from 9 to 11 A.M..

Ludwig Mann was one of Alzheimer's closest co-workers; he taught a practical course on the diagnosis and treatment of nervous illnesses and presented many patients. His special fields were nervous disorders and electrodiagnosis.

Another colleague was Ottfried Förster, a well-known representative of the Breslau school, a neurologist, neurosurgeon, and psychiatrist of world renown who distinguished himself at congresses in Germany and abroad through his remarkable lectures. In his home town of Breslau, Förster gave a lecture with the aid of photographs and film. A contemporary witness aptly described this event:

From then on, however, he became the master photographer of neurology. The image [Förster's] of how he holds and directs the patients, like an artist his cello, stayed with us in so many ways. Never again was the everyday and the fullness of life in the finely contoured, still youthful face so uninterruptedly happy as at that time.[4]

Alzheimer was also fascinated by his colleague's lecture, and Förster valued Alzheimer's scientific contributions, which had already gained attention in Munich through didactic presentations using the new projection system, and supported his appointment in Breslau.

Many years later—after Alzheimer's death—Förster was sent to Russia at the request of the Foreign Office to treat the critically ill, hemiparetic, and aphasic Lenin. Förster quickly gained the patient's trust. After hours of conversation he was fascinated by Lenin's extraordinary mental powers, his quick perception, his precise thought, and his matter-of-fact outlook. Until Lenin's death in January 1924, Förster remained his personal physician.

Georg Stertz also was among Alzheimer's close co-workers. Stertz gave lectures in neurology, general psychiatry, and the history of psychiatry; he also gave practical lessons with demonstrations for doctors and jurists. Furthermore, he was responsible for practical training in histology and directed the institute laboratory.

Stertz was born and raised in Breslau and completed his medical studies there, becoming a doctor in 1903. After periods at the Eppendorf Clinic in Hamburg and the Pathology Institute in Freiburg he was again in Eppendorf for two years from 1904 to 1906 as an intern under Max Nonne, a famous neurologist after whom Nonne–Marie disease, an atrophy of the nerve cells in the brain stem, is named.

In 1907 Stertz became an intern at the Breslau Psychiatric Clinic under Alzheimer's predecessor, Karl Bonhoeffer; in 1910 he moved to the Psychiatric Clinic in Bonn under Alexander Westphal, who together with Wilhelm Erb had described the absence or weakening of the patellar reflex, the Erb–Westphal sign. Stertz completed his *Habilitation* in Bonn in 1911, and in 1912 Alzheimer brought the thirty-four-year-old back to Breslau, later appointing him chief physician and, in 1914, unsalaried professor.

Stertz, who later married Alzheimer's daughter, found that Alzheimer fulfilled his duties with an incredible thoroughness. He described him as a physician in the best and noblest sense of the word, a doctor and humanitarian who offered his patients not only his great experience and skill but also his heart.

Alzheimer built up an atmosphere of kindness and humanity that, as many of his former patients affirmed, left behind an unforgettable impression. However, he was also extraordinarily critical of himself and others and placed the greatest value on honesty, diligence, and conscientiousness.

He was polite, sincere, and helpful to his assistants and students in the clinic and the laboratory, but only when he was convinced that this cooperation was in the interest of the clinic and of science and only as long as he saw in the co-worker an unconditional love for scientific truth.

If he noticed the slightest violation of this principle—and his interns and chief physicians could remember this well—he felt wounded and acted in an unexpectedly stringent manner.

Although the teaching load made heavy demands on Alzheimer's time, he was constantly present in the clinic and examined many patients himself. On November 18, 1912, he carefully elicited the medical history of a twenty-seven-year-old governess:

> Her speech was striking for its slowness and affectedness. Her siblings teased her because of it, but she gave the excuse that she could no longer speak any other way. Soon afterward ensued complaints of weakness and pains in the left arm and frequent vomiting. After a while a stiffness in her gait became noticeable. She was depressed, with an inclination to crying that from time to time assumed a convulsive character. She first entered a sanatorium and then Prof. Mann's private clinic. From there she was finally transferred to the psychiatric clinic.
>
> The patient appeared completely rational and oriented at the time of admission but did not want to recall the trip home from London to Germany. She had supposedly last had pains in her left arm in April, which, she said, had rapidly increased in intensity. After treatment in the sanatorium she claimed a temporary improvement but then a progressive worsening of the condition.
>
> When she speaks, she said, she gets a cramp in her arm. She claimed to have avoided all speech for a while for this reason. She often curtseys with the left foot. She easily swallows the wrong

way and sometimes apparently gets food up her nose. Cries easily but also returns quickly to a cheerful mood.[5]

Then a professional debate developed when on February 13, 1913, Stertz presented the patient under the auspices of a meeting of the Breslau Psychiatric–Neurological Association. Stertz thought the patient was hysterical. Prof. Ludwig Mann, on the other hand, assumed an organic disorder with comorbid hysterical symptoms.

C. S. Freund, a co-worker at Alzheimer's clinic, saw the painful muscle cramps as catalyzed by a mild inflammation of the nerves.

In contrast, Alzheimer and neurosurgeon Ottfriend Förster argued that a disease of the brain and spinal cord could not catalyze such a condition. Alzheimer stated, "An organic disease is unimaginable. Clinical observation points to a strong psychogenic suggestibility." He therefore assumed hysteria.

On May 20, 1913, epileptic attacks occurred, and the patient's temperature climbed to 41.8 degrees Celsius. On May 22, 1913, she died at 7:45 A.M. in a deep stupor, without any signs of further convulsions. As a result, Alzheimer remarked, "Even if there could now be no doubt that an organic condition lay at the basis of the clinical picture, it still appeared quite impossible to classify it with any known illness," and then he admitted to the diagnostic uncertainty in this case. He confessed self-critically that "our anatomic and physiological knowledge is burdened with countless gaps, which can for this reason easily lead us to erroneous conclusions."

The medical history of the patient appeared to Alzheimer so remarkable that he decided to publish it under the title "On a Peculiar Disease of the Central Nervous System with Bulbar Syndromes and Painful Spastic Convulsions of the Extremities." Alzheimer's health did not allow him to complete this essay; the manuscript was found among his papers.

His successor in Munich, Walter Spielmeyer, published the essay posthumously and commented in a footnote, "This work was clearly complete in the essentials. We could limit ourselves to minor corrections of the parts of the dictation that Alzheimer had not yet revised. The illustrations probably were intended to be text figures. Several pictures that were supposed to illustrate the general topography of the medulla oblongata could not be found, but the description in the text still produces an overview of the distribution of the lesions, so that nothing need be regarded as lost with these pictures for the overall representation."

All in all, 1913 was very eventful. Although he was severely ill, Alzheimer continued to give lectures and write essays.

Under the auspices of the Breslau Psychiatric–Neurologic Organization in February 1913 he gave several lectures and appeared a total of three times, speaking about peculiar metasyphilitic diseases (that is, illnesses that manifest themselves after a long-lasting syphilis) and hallucinoses. Afterward he spoke on late epilepsy and gave an account of a distinctive condition of stupor with an arteriosclerotic basis. His chief physicians were also active at this event and made valuable contributions.

One can infer from the minutes of the meetings that Alzheimer was a lively and critical discussant. After his lecture on a "peculiar metasyphilitic disease" at the meeting on February 17, 1913, he decisively rejected the suggestion that a brain puncture be carried out solely for diagnostic purposes in view of the accompanying dangers: "Such a risky intervention can be justified only when therapeutic interventions would be made possible by the result of the aspiration." He justified his position with a case of stupor that occurred after a brain puncture.[6]

After this conference, Alzheimer had reached the limit of his strength. His friends convinced him to take a cure, and at the end of February 1913 he telephoned his renowned Wiesbaden colleague Dr. Abend, a specialist in internal medicine, who ran a private clinic in Wiesbaden's finest location, Parkstrasse 30. The decision to go to the private clinic Villa Luna, a special clinic for gastrointestinal illnesses, appears dubious today because insofar as one can diagnose it retrospectively, Alzheimer appears to have had a serious heart condition.

The train journey passed without complications. In the elegant health resort town, "the traveler is awaited by a metropolitan fleet of carriages, from the simplest one-horse hackney carriage to luxurious two-horse equipage, to carry him to the desired hotel," as the Wiesbaden health resort prospectus promises. "By means of an exemplarily executed and officially supervised order any jostling in going to the carriages is avoided. A set fee regulates the price so that the stranger is protected from cheating."

Alzheimer had himself driven from the monumental train station to "one of the most beautiful and best-equipped health spas in Germany" in a two-horse carriage down Wilhelmstrasse, an extremely elegant, boulevard-like strip, past the splendid spa grounds of the Warm Damm to Dr. Abend's private clinic on Parkstrasse.

On Sunday, March 23, 1913, Alzheimer's name appeared in supplement No. 82 of the *Wiesbaden Bade-Blatt* cure-list of March 20: "Alzheimer, Mr. Univ.-Prof. Dr. Med., Breslau, health resort Dr. Abend," and the same entry appeared on March 30, 1913. When the Lord Mayor of Wiesbaden, Karl von Ibell, officially opened the Kaiser Friedrich Spa on March 25, 1913, Alzheimer had the opportunity to undergo the modern treatment offered by the so-called Wiesbaden cure.

Fifty thermal baths with twenty-five rooms for resting; mud and carbonic acid baths; electro-, heat, and hydrotherapy; fango packs (therapeutic mud packs); and especially the electrical heat therapy devices developed by Dr. Türnauer reflected the latest therapeutic techniques.

During his time at the resort Alzheimer was visited by Franz Nissl: "In 1913 I visited him in Wiesbaden, where he was receiving medical treatment because of his heart complaint. When he came to Heidelberg on his way home, I could inwardly be very pleased about his recovery. . . . But he did not want to hear about conserving his strength, and wanted instead to keep going for as long as he could."[7] Nissl's next visit with Alzheimer, in Heidelberg, was his last.

Shortly before Alzheimer's departure, his daughter Maria arrived in Wiesbaden and brought family gossip with her: His chief physician, Georg Stertz, and Alzheimer's daughter Gertrud had fallen in love.

The generous father put Maria up in one of the best houses in town, a "hotel with its own thermal waters," the *Kaiserbad* on the opulent Wilhelmstrasse, and spent a few days with her in this health resort town, one of the most elegant of the time of the *Jugendstil*, or art nouveau movement. Maria stayed for several more weeks in Wiesbaden, as one can infer from the *Wiesbaden Bade-Blatt* of April 13, 1913.

At the same time, in the Hotel Vier Jahreszeiten (Four Seasons) on Kaiser Friedrichplatz were lodged some very grand personages: "Her Highness the Princess-Mother of Schaumburg-Lippe, Duchess of Saxony and retinue; Court-Martial Chamberlain von Kaisenberg, Court Lady Freiin von Toll and servants, Bückeburg," "His Lordship Highness Prince Friedrich Christian of Schaumburg-Lippe with entourage, Bückeburg," and "Her Ladyship Highness Princess Elisabeth of Schaumburg-Lippe with entourage, Bückeburg."[8]

Back in Breslau, stronger but not cured, Alzheimer set to work on the next task, the meeting of the German Association for Psychiatry in May 1913, at which he would give a lecture on the pathological anatomy of dementia praecox, or schizophrenia. As editor of the *Zeitschrift für die Gesamte Neurologie und Psychiatrie* (*Journal of Complete Neurology and Psychiatry*) he used the opportunity to publish several articles on the same theme.

In 1913 an extensive work, "25 Years of Psychiatry: A Retrospective on the Occasion of the 25th Anniversary of Prof. Dr. Emil Sioli as director of the Frankfurt Mental Asylum," was published in the respected *Archiv für Psychiatrie*. The publication begins,

> Twenty-five years ago Prof. Dr. Sioli took over the position as director of the Municipal Mental Asylum at Frankfurt. Among the many burdens that Sioli's office brought him twenty-five years ago was the task of introducing the author of these lines to psychiatry. I worked under him for the first fourteen years of his activity in Frankfurt. I was permitted to see how he transformed a strange asylum into his own and to help him with it, and more than any of his other students I can testify to what he accomplished.
>
> Quietly effective and averse to too much writing, through his writings he gives only a very incomplete picture of his comprehensive work. Many thoughts that others later wrote down and carried out we, his students, had already heard him express or seen him put into action. For twenty-five years he has contributed with a tireless passion to the progress of psychiatry.

Alzheimer had only praise for his old boss and in the last sentence of the publication expressed the wish that "an internal relationship between research and practice would gradually open up in psychiatry, which we today often miss and which would certainly benefit to both sides and would make possible a more rapid solution of the tasks that we face in the next twenty-five years."

A few months after the meeting of the German Association for Psychiatry, Alzheimer was host of the annual conference of the Society of German Doctors of Nervous Disease, which took place in Breslau from September 29 to October 1, 1913. He was very active and participated with two contributions of his own: He spoke about a process of degeneration in the nervous system and demonstrated on a series of brains and brain sections two different kinds of developmental inhibition, macrogyria and microgyria (in which the cerebral convolutions are too big or too small, respectively). These cases were published directly afterward in his house journal.

Kraepelin, who attended this congress, noticed that Alzheimer was no longer the man he had known in Munich: "In 1913 I saw him again in Breslau at the conference of German Doctors of Nervous Disease. Although his outward appearance was sprightly, his mood was dejected and depressed; he looked into the future with bleak foreboding. It was our last meeting. In the effort to perform his duties fully, Alzheimer did not take proper care of himself."[9]

The many demands of everyday life at the clinic and the routine administrative details took their toll on Alzheimer's health. Several documented examples show the kinds of administrative and technical problems with which Alzheimer struggled. He reported to the university registrar on June 11, 1913, about two scientific discoveries of importance to psychiatry and neurology: proof of the syphilis pathogen in the brain and spinal cord in general paresis and atrophy of the spinal cord, and the serologic method founded by Emil Abderhalden, which would be drawn on in the diagnosis of mental illnesses.

Alzheimer regarded it as his duty to introduce this method of examination into his clinic "so that both methods of early recognition and diagnosis of mental illnesses could be called upon and can contribute to success in therapy."[10] He therefore applied for funding to purchase the necessary equipment, which was approved on July 21, 1913.

Two of Alzheimer's research activities from 1914 are of interest. On May 27, 1914, he had to oversee the screening of patients from other asylums in the province.

On June 9, 1914, he applied to the Royal Ministry of Justice in Berlin to produce a questionnaire for the royal penal institutions that was supposed to provide information about German patients who had been members of the French Foreign Legion: "Because cases accumulate in which former Foreign Legionnaires are admitted to psychiatric clinics because of psychological illnesses, it would be desirable to understand the corresponding forms of mental disturbance that motivate entry into the French Foreign Legion," whereby he argued that it was important "to get insight into the personality and the social milieu of the patients."

But issues of scientific significance were not always at stake; mundane details also occupied his time. On June 15, 1914, he applied for permission for

1. Covering of radiators in the unit for unruly patients
2. Venetian sunblinds for the lending library on the top floor
3. A warmer floor for the porter's ground floor recreation room, which gets very cold in winter
4. The improvement, and, relatedly, renewal of the paint on the beds and other furniture
5. The acquisition of a bookshelf, writing desk, and two tooth-brush cupboards in the patient units
6. Better comfort for the rooms of private patients, e.g., better seating, beds, and pillows
7. Linoleum covering on sixty worn-out dessert dishes
8. Replacement of the bell signal in sick rooms with a light signal so as not to disturb the calm patients, who are very much in need of rest

The clinic's budget ran to a total of 3649.20 marks. A request to pay 1000 marks to a laboratory assistant who was responsible for brain sections was rejected in June 1914. At this point, everyone had other concerns.

The World War had begun.


## Psychiatry in a Time of War

The shots in Sarajevo that murdered the Austro-Hungarian heirs apparent on June 28, 1914, precipitated World War I.

While young men were drawn into battle with cries of "Hurrah!" the voices of warning were stifled by cries of treason. Alzheimer's son, Hans, who had been a member of the Marian congregation since 1912, a school group that met for common prayer and meditation, left boarding school and volunteered for the cavalry, which pleased his father.

The war marked not only world events but also the fates of individual people, very directly, in both private and professional life. On November 6, 1914, Alzheimer attended an evening meeting on war medicine for the medical section of the Silesian Society for Patriotic Culture and reported on several cases of methyl alcohol poisoning of soldiers, some with fatal outcomes, and gave a lecture called "Fatal Effects of the War on the Nervous System and Psyche."[11]

In Alzheimer's private list of publications, the work on the cases of methyl alcohol poisoning was cited as number 52. A further lecture that Alzheimer gave to "The Best of the Breslau National Women's Service as a War Lecture of the Breslau University Lecturers 1915" has also been preserved. The accompanying publication, "War and the Nerves," is one of his last, and it is particularly worth reading and typical of Alzheimer's work at this time.[12]

Alzheimer initially presented himself as a brain researcher:

When we subject to scrutiny the connections between the war and the nerves, we think less of the nerves in the narrow sense, those white strands that run from the brain and spinal cord through the body to the sensory organs, skin, muscles, and joints like wires to transmit sensations to the brain or impulses of the will to the muscles, and more of the nervous central organ, especially the brain, the organ of our soul, in which thinking, feeling, and acting has its seat.

Extraordinarily intricate in its construction, composed of countless cells of the most diverse forms, which are bound together again in an infinite variety of ways through the finest nerve threads, it represents a form of complexity like no other that creative nature has produced. To it we owe the possibility of human culture. When we talk about tough nerves, a courageous heart, or cold blood, what we are really talking about are achievements of the brain.

Then Alzheimer turned to his real theme: "Courage and intrepidity, endurance and bravery, the ability to sacrifice oneself, and comradeship are soldierly virtues that are bound up with our brain's accomplishments. Certainly the soldier needs healthy limbs, strong muscles, good lungs, and a properly functioning heart, but those are just tools, tools that are able to achieve something outstanding only under the command of the brain."

At this point the scientifically inclined lecture took a turn that reveals that he could not escape the general mood of the time:

However, the war places special demands not only on the nerves of the soldiers but also on those of everyone who has to remain at home; that is something that we can observe in ourselves. That August day lay itself upon our nerves as heavily as a lead weight, when the war had become a matter of fact.

For decades we had lived quietly and safely, and nothing appeared to prevent us from harvesting the fruits of our peaceful labor in future years. But at a single blow everything became uncertain: the fate of our brothers, sons, and friends, whom we saw mobilized—indeed, the future of the entire family.

We hoped for a decisive victory, but who could have told us then that an enemy out to kill would not break into our homes, scorch our cities, and ravage our fields? And what if we have deluded ourselves in our hopes? The fatherland was threatened from all sides, and we knew only too well that we could expect no protection if we did not triumph.

An inner unease seized hold of most people. Who could still sit there quietly among his books or devote himself to quiet work? How small, how meaningless that all at once appeared against that one thing: what the next day would bring. One ran after every new newspaper, waited impatiently for every special edition.

Alzheimer became frankly militant: "We must contribute again and again everything that we possess of strong nerves and cultivate the soldierly virtues that the poets have always praised so brilliantly, which we hardly find the opportunity to practice during peacetime."

In light of this view it is understandable why Alzheimer's son, Hans, barely eighteen years old, volunteered and participated in the war. Many doctors, including Stertz, who in the meantime had grown much closer to Alzheimer's daughter Gertrud, marched into battle, and Alzheimer— flanked by innumerable yet insufficient medical aides—had to manage a sudden avalanche of incoming clinic admissions and requests for expert assessments. A Breslau colleague reported, "Despite his increasing health complaints Alzheimer subjected himself to this new workload for an entire year, not even avoiding the frequent strains of outside court appointments." And another colleague and contemporary witness remarked, "The pressure of war work weighed heavily on Alzheimer, and the illness had already cast a shadow on his personality and brought about a strange irritability in his otherwise essentially happy nature."

In the publication "War and the Nerves" Alzheimer also described the behavior of the people who remained behind: "People fearful by nature, who were then overcome by rash fear and saw everything in black, packed their suitcases, left, and then returned, in order to pack up yet again at the next alarming report from the east."

He wrote about the emergence of rumors: "Before an official war report had something to announce, chatterboxes, both male and female, eagerly spread adventurous rumors about colossal victories or appreciable losses. Every new mouth that repeated the story increased the scale of the victory or defeat and had heard the report from a 'trustworthy source.'"

Alzheimer also saw the "spy hunt" and the attacks on armored cars in the first August days as signs of emotion clouding judgment. "The entire war mood and the unsettling feeling of being threatened made one see spies in every conspicuous or foreign-looking character, that is, people whom we today could not regard as suspicious. Nor was it only the usual rowdy public on the street; rather, more serious people also could be seen to participate in an often violent way in their persecution and exposure."

About the problem of panic buying he said, "Signs of a similar kind were disclosed in the runs on the savings banks and the food stores in the first days of the war. The authorities had to make a serious call for calm until the hustle and bustle reached an end."

Alongside these signs, interesting for a general psychology of the *Volk*, Alzheimer then described the actual psychological harm that could be observed as an effect of the war. The thoroughness with which Alzheimer described the individual clinical pictures could have come from a comprehensive textbook of war psychiatry.

Alzheimer mentioned severe mental disorders, "which stand in a certain, if clearly only loose connection," and spoke about melancholy and especially about melancholy women, who despaired because the deaths of so many soldiers took away from them any hope of marriage. He also depicted the case of a woman who stubbornly refused to eat with the justification that she did not want to eat up and take from others what little remained.

Alzheimer recognized with acumen that swindlers and soldiers, who have always had a flair for imaginative life, could now live out these inclinations: "Here and there surfaced a young man, hardly ripe for military service, who told the story of how, because of some outstanding service or other that he had performed in the field, he had earned a higher military rank . . . and that then Hindenburg, the Crown Prince, or the Kaiser had especially praised him or had invited him to his table. . . . One knows these 'Tartarins of Tarascon' [a kind of show-off; a figure of French writer Alphonse Daudet] in psychiatry as pathological liars, hysterical swindlers, or *Pseudologica Phantastica.*"

Alzheimer explored the psychological troubles of soldiers and established that "it is the impression of every working psychiatrist that the number of milder psychological disorders, the so-called nervous ones, have increased to a substantial degree." These psychological disorders he divided into those that can be traced to external causes and those based on a particular disposition and heredity.

In conclusion, he described the mood-elevating effect of alcohol, to which he attributed an important role in the causation of mental disorders.

Alzheimer also regarded the emergence and course of other mental illnesses, including general paresis, from the perspective of the war. By this time it was known that general paresis was a consequence of syphilis. In relation to the war Alzheimer commented, "The number of cases that have been observed during the war does not appear to be very large; in some the first signs of illness certainly manifest themselves before the soldiers are sent into combat." Concerning so-called exhaustion neurasthenia of soldiers, Alzheimer saw promising signs of rapid recovery: "Several weeks of rest and good nutrition usually suffice to regain complete readiness for service."

To Alzheimer, of greater importance than the wartime mental illnesses caused by external factors were those that originate in disposition and heredity. "Of them, youthful conditions of stupefaction and so-called manic–depressive insanity are of the most practical importance because they provide the largest number of patients who must be cared for in the mental asylums. Naturally we also see these frequent illnesses among the soldiers, who represent a substantial segment of the entire population. However, nothing suggests that they appear during war in larger numbers."

He observed that during war epileptic seizures are especially common after severe physical and mental strains. Alzheimer also had something to say about hysteria:

We can regard it as a quite special characteristic of hysteria that mental impressions of an excitational kind can cause psychological or even manifold physical disorders with extraordinary ease.

Thus we see, for example, that when in wartime a grenade explodes in direct proximity to a soldier he can lose speech or hearing or both, that is, become a deaf–mute, without being hit by shrapnel or even being injured, in other words solely as a result of the violent fright. He can also show paralysis in both legs or one half of his body; convulsions can set in; a stupor can develop, a dreamlike, depressed condition of consciousness in which the patient is disoriented about place and time and confused in all sorts of ways. In such states patients often produce statements tied to or standing in some relation to the experience of fright.

Alzheimer commented as follows on the severe psychological shock effects that appear after battles:

Sometimes we succeed here in clearing up serious paralyses through a powerful suggestion: Stand up and walk! Having developed as the result of psychological influences, the paralyses can also be alleviated with their help. Mostly, however, it takes a longer period of continual psychological influence supported by all kinds of medication to clear away the signs of illness.

Apart from these classic mental illnesses, the effects of which were for the most part amplified by the war, Alzheimer also observed something completely new, which he called *Rentenneurose* (pension neurosis):

Closely related to these disorders are those in which a slight wound, such as a graze from a bullet or a fall from a horse or a carriage, binds together a bunch of subjective complaints for which an examination of the nervous system finds no foundation and which stand in absolutely no relation to the trivial injury. It is not at all rare that we see these disorders in peacetime in workers who have had an accident on the job and in people who have survived a railroad accident, and we designate them traumatic hysteria or pension neuroses because it can probably be justly believed that the anticipation of a pension is the psychological factor that maintains the symptoms.

Alzheimer even made a congenital defect responsible for this pension-desiring behavior: "It is the so-called degenerates, psychopaths, or inferiors. Often we are dealing here with the children of the mentally ill, of epileptics, criminals, or drinkers. . . . Often they sign on as volunteers; however, what attracts them often is only the uniform and the attractive exterior. But the initial inspiration is gone with the first difficulties."

He continued, "When the International Congress for Mental Health Care met several years ago in Berlin, the military medical expert opinion on these degenerates was on the agenda. French, Russian, English, and German psychiatrists all agreed that they were to be kept away from military service as much as possible because they harmed the morale and discipline of the troops."

It is astonishing that Alzheimer expressed himself so firmly about this phenomenon, although he had no reliable reports on susceptibility to such mental illnesses in either the German or the enemy armies. There were at most newspaper reports, which themselves were based on unreliable sources.

Thus one reads in the newspapers of an increasing number of mental illnesses appearing in the trenches in Flanders among the British troops as well as parts of the British colonial army, and it was also reported that in the Russian army numerous mental disorders arose, namely, that the soldiers had seen visions of the Mother of God, who had apparently promised them imminent peace.

Alzheimer somewhat carelessly took all of this at face value when in his optimistic way he said, "If in conclusion we look back again, then first of all we see . . . that even in war a person with a healthy nervous system is in very little danger of becoming mentally ill."

Had he lived to see the end of World War I he might have regretted the following words:

Yes, we may even devote ourselves to the confident expectation
that the war, which inflicts some wounds on the nerves, also creates its uses for them. . . . The war also trains a more determined,
daring, enterprising race.

With strengthened nerves the German *Volk* will then embark
on the tasks of peace that the future will place before it and also
be well able to master the many symptoms that a long period of
peace allows to grow rampant and which some overly concerned
people have regarded as proof of a psychological degeneration of
our *Volk*.

## Alzheimer's Death

By 1915 Alzheimer constantly had to attend to his health and take longer
pauses to recover during almost all activities, a circumstance completely
unknown to him in earlier days.

In arranging the wedding of his eldest daughter, Gertrud, to Stertz in
May 1915, he had to summon the last ounce of his strength. The wedding
was celebrated with an Alzheimerian splendor, with many friends and colleagues as guests. However, his illness was increasingly apparent to both
friends and outsiders. Gaupp, above all, could not help but notice: "In fall
1915, when I visited him for the last time in Breslau, he confessed with the
quiet courage, great also in suffering, that was his nature, that he was not
well and that he would probably soon have to place the care of his children
in the hands of his siblings and his son-in-law." And although he could feel
that his end was near, his optimism and humor continued to remain as con-
vincingly apparent as in earlier days.

Gaupp documented several of their last conversations, in which
Alzheimer remembered the many co-workers from abroad in the Munich
anatomy laboratory: "They will want to come back after the war! I don't
believe that they will avoid me as a barbarian, because they never had to
complain about me."[13]

He called himself a "barbarian" ironically, in contrast to his sensitive
and noble-looking Italian guest doctors in Munich, alongside whom his ex-
uberant manner occasionally appeared somewhat crude. After a particularly successful drawing of slide preparations with the camera lucida, he often
gave his colleagues a powerful clap on the shoulders.

Alzheimer increasingly suffered from agonizing chest pains; nevertheless, he did not slow down. At this time he was interested in the theme of
idiocy and planned a treatment of it, but the project did not get beyond the

planning stage. In October he became bedridden; at the end of November kidney failure set in, with growing shortness of breath. The title of Cabinet councillor (*Geheimer Ministerialrat*) was conferred upon him; because of his constantly changing state of awareness it was unclear whether he could grasp the fact that he had received the honor.

Georg Stertz obtained a leave of absence from the field—he was in Spa on the Western Front—and arrived in Breslau in the first week of December, concerned about his father-in-law's health.

Gaupp checked in now and then by telephone from Tübingen to inquire after Alzheimer's health and wrote some affectionate letters. He received a reply from Stertz dated December 12, 1915, a few days before Alzheimer's death, in which Stertz first thanked Gaupp in the name of the family for his sympathetic letter:

Unfortunately I have only bad news to report on the state of my father-in-law's health. In the last week or so there has been a rather rapid decline of his powers, and his consciousness has also become increasingly cloudy, and from time to time he is quite delirious. His shortness of breath was lasting and strong, and has only recently eased somewhat, so that now, at least, his subjective suffering is not so bad. We are assuming an unchanging condition, and the hope that there will be another improvement has fallen away.

I very much fear that the family will lose its beloved father and I, at the same time, my spiritual leader forever. In these hard days we have all become convinced that death will come as a redeemer. In his last episode of complete mental clarity Papa had the great joy of seeing his Hans, who had suddenly arrived for a fourteen-day vacation. He was so happy and grateful to be able to see him and speak to him again. I myself was deeply saddened and sometimes quite desolate that I had not been able to relieve my father-in-law of work and strain during a hard time for him, where some relief could still have been of real use.

While I was in Spa and hardly able to use half of my strength, I repeatedly requested urgently that he have me called back. Unfortunately, he decided to do that only at the last moment, when it was no longer practicable, and then another substantial delay was caused by an error in official channels. I had to be content to free him recently from the pressure of breathing difficulties and to stand a little by him, my wife, and the family in this most serious of times as well as I could. I am very sorry that I cannot give you better news.

I hope your youngest is in good health again and can look forward with his siblings, whom of course I also know in part, to the approaching Christmas. Indeed, the children are so happy about it that they do not notice anything of the cares of the time, and of course despite everything we would not at all want to miss having experienced with full awareness our country's poverty and war. Everyone at home, especially Gertrud, sends their greetings to you, and I include myself in the hope that you transfer a little of the friendship you feel for the Alzheimer family to me.[14]

On Sunday, December 19, 1915, death seemed imminent. Around Alzheimer's deathbed assembled Gertrud and Georg Stertz, Alzheimer's nineteen-year-old son, Hans, and fifteen-year-old Maria. Alzheimer's sister Elisabeth, the constantly loyal Maja, who had already witnessed Cecilie's death, was also present. At age fifty-one Alois Alzheimer died, surrounded by his family.

After his death an unusually strong sympathy found expression in the many death notices that appeared in the *Schlesischen Zeitung* (*Silesian News*) on Tuesday, December 21.[15]

The family and the "deeply mourning bereaved" announced,

Tonight after a long and serious illness our dear father, father-in-law, and brother gently passed away, the full professor in the medical faculty and director of the Royal Psychiatric Clinic Dr. Alois Alzheimer at the age of not yet fifty-two years.

Breslau, December 19, 1915

Auenstrasse 42

The funeral will take place quietly in Frankfurt.

Flowers gratefully declined.

The rector and senate of the Silesian Friedrich-Wilhelm University in Breslau paid tribute to the deceased as follows:

Imbued with deep sorrow we announce the sad tidings of the departure of the full professor in the medical faculty and director of the psychiatric clinic Dr. Alois Alzheimer, who on the morning of December 19 fell victim to a pernicious illness at the age of fifty-one years.

In the deceased medical science loses one of its best, a researcher distinguished by profound works; the unhappy army of people shattered by madness and nervous illness loses a paternally concerned and skilled caretaker; the sick bay loses a friend to soldiers, one inflamed by ideals and by his selfless conception of his difficult calling.

His scientific reputation, which he had already gained as chief physician at the Municipal Mental Asylum in Frankfurt (1888–1903) as well as a scientific assistant at the psychiatric clinics in Heidelberg and Munich (1903 to 1912), he fully consolidated through his exemplary teaching activity and direction of the psychiatric clinic at our university. Although he moved in our circles for only three years, he won the hearts of all his colleagues and students through his natural openness and rectitude and through his complete devotion to the calling of academic teaching. We will preserve the respectful memory of this dear colleague always.

The assistants at the clinic commemorated their director in their own notice:

During the night from Saturday to Sunday Prof. Dr. Alois Alzheimer passed away after many weeks of illness. We lose in him not only our highly esteemed teacher, who will always remain a shining example to us in our scientific work and in the loyal fulfillment of our medical duties, but also and above all a truly fatherly friend whose memory we will never forget.

Sick bay inspector deputy Hoffmann found the following words:

On December 19, 1915, Prof. Dr. Alois Alzheimer, the leading doctor of the Fortress sick bay Breslau, Royal Psychiatric Clinic unit, passed away after long illness. The memory of this universally revered deceased will be held in high honor by me and the medical teams and noncommissioned officers in service in the unit.

The medical faculty of the Silesian Friedrich-Wilhelm University expressed its mourning:

The medical faculty announces with deep sorrow the departure of its member, the full professor of psychiatry and neurology Dr. Alzheimer. Through the winning way of his unusually sympathetic personality, his devotion to the teaching duties he had undertaken, his creative power and the depths of his scientific works, and, not least of all, through his selfless and noble view of his medical calling he became a model of the academic teacher. He carried out his tasks during wartime with the purest enthusiasm. Although these tasks doubled with his work in the sick bays, he bore them with superhuman strength until a destructive illness put a premature end to his idealistic striving. In the history of the psychiatric clinic of our faculty his name and works will live on in perpetuity.

The head doctor of the fortress sick bay, Senior Registrar Scholz, paid him tribute thus:

After serious illness, Dr. Alois Alzheimer, professor at the Silesian Friedrich-Wilhelm University and director of the psychiatric clinic (Fortress sick bay unit), died yesterday. Since the beginning of the war the deceased devoted every ounce of his strength to the fatherland and through his substantial knowledge and ability proved of invaluable service to the Fortress sick bay, which ensures the dearly departed a lasting, honorable memory.

Finally, his loyal co-workers also published a notice:

Tonight our highly esteemed boss, Prof. Dr. Alois Alzheimer, director of the Royal Psychiatric Clinic, died. Those who knew him will mourn our terrible loss.

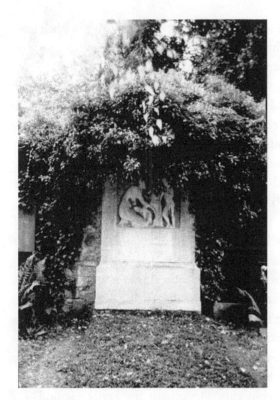

FIGURE 6.2 *The grave site of Cecilie and Alois Alzheimer at the main cemetery in Frankfurt am Main*

On December 23, 1915, Alois Alzheimer was quietly laid to rest next to his wife, Cecilie. His old friend Nissl accompanied the family: "As quietly and simply as his life expired, so modest too was his burial. He had requested that a speech be made at the gravesite. On December 23 we accompanied our friend to his last resting place."[16]

Alzheimer now rested at the side of his beloved Cecilie and among illustrious people, quite close to the ancestors of his wife, who found their final rest in the Jewish part of the cemetery. Later, writer Ricarda Huch was buried close by; Huch was born in the same year as Alzheimer and died, well advanced in years, in 1947.

The Bethmanns, well-known Frankfurt bankers, benefactors, donors, founders, and supporters of the arts and sciences, have their family tomb in the vicinity. In 1918 Ludwig Erdinger found his final rest there; Paul Ehrlich, who, like Alzheimer, died in 1915, was buried in the Jewish part of the cemetery, as were the Rothschilds. Other psychiatrists can be found there: Heinrich Hoffmann and his predecessor, Johann Georg Varrentrapp.

The sculptor family Klimsch, one of whom had made the Alzheimers' gravestone, has its tomb there, not far from Feuerbach's grave and that of philosopher Arthur Schopenhauer.

As quiet as proceedings were at his grave, the obituaries that appeared in many psychiatric specialty journals in 1916 were passionate and full of praise. Clemens Neisser's obituary, which he presented as a lecture on December 9, 1916, at the conference of the Eastern German Association for Psychiatry, can be regarded as both the most fitting and the most sincere. Neisser, at that time a well-known psychiatrist and director of the asylum in Lublinitz, paid tribute to Alzheimer in the following way:

> Since last we assembled, our association has suffered serious losses. First among them stands the bitter blow that struck us with the death of our chair, Prof. Alzheimer, who almost a year ago, on December 19, 1915, succumbed to the illness that overcame him when he traveled here to Breslau, here to the goal of a new, independent mode of working and teaching in this outstanding location, after he had already long earned his place in the scientific world through his work as a researcher.
>
> Gentlemen! The obituaries throughout the entire medical world give a picture of the outstanding importance of Alzheimer and, in particular, of the warm respect that was paid to his character as a researcher and a man. I am not able to say anything new to you, nothing better than, to name just a few, Landowsky, who found such fine words, or our colleague Stertz, who had the good fortune to become so especially close to the deceased during his work here, and Spielmeyer, who so masterfully depicted Alzheimer's life's work with the piety of a student.
>
> For the closer circle of our association, only two meetings of which he attended, Alzheimer's work naturally could not, in its direct effect, mean the same as that of his predecessors, in particular that of the unforgettable Wernicke and of Bonhoeffer. . . .
>
> Nevertheless, in the meeting of December 7, 1912, at which he became a member of our association, he immediately led us into his very own field of work in his lecture "On a Still Not Precisely Known, Paresis-Like Clinical Picture," and through his suggestions in relation to the treatment of general paresis he prompted

common action in the clinic and the provincial asylums from this position so that we might hope for closer scientific cooperation and for support of our own work.

That Alzheimer was outstanding and irreplaceable as an anatomic–histologic brain researcher was emphasized—in the obituaries and memorial speeches too—from all sides. But I believe that one can do justice to his special importance only when one bears in mind that Alzheimer embraced clinical questions with at least an equal interest and that he constantly kept them in mind during his anatomic work, without ever disregarding the independence of each field of research or failing to recognize the limits that could be reached in connecting their separate results.

Precisely this fact appears to me to be of special importance for our view of Alzheimer's scientific development and his success as a researcher. It explains why Alzheimer entered into a closer relationship with Kraepelin's school—inwardly as well—than did Wernicke, despite his more anatomic way of thinking.

In Frankfurt Alzheimer, with all of the tools of refined technology, which he mastered as few do, even participating for years in their development, could well accomplish fruitful work and define his field's perspectives with the unerring clarity characteristic of him. It was thanks to the directness and simplicity of his way of posing questions, in conjunction with the painstaking reliability of his working methods, that he, as far as I know, never had to retract or take back anything that he had published as a scientific result.

In Alzheimer existed an unusually happy mixture of optimistic confidence regarding the achievability of scientific goals and cautious skepticism regarding all individual results. And with these characteristics, which were the foundation of his fame as a researcher, mingled an unusual mastery of the word and an ability to give well-rounded didactic presentations, which made his lectures a pleasure and ensured that his remarks in discussion always had an effect.

If I may be permitted to add something personal, then let me say that I remember with gratitude the friendly relationship that involved me with Alzheimer for more than twenty years, and I remember with particular pleasure the visit that he made to me in the middle of the 1890s in Leubus. But the hopes that I had placed in closer personal contact with him then have not been fulfilled.

The pressure of war work weighed heavily on Alzheimer, and the illness had already thrown a shadow across his character and brought about an otherwise foreign irritability in his essentially happy nature. But those who could not compare, who did not know him before, still fell completely under the spell of this gifted, strong, and kind personality, and I am sure that you, gentlemen, that we will all have a reverential, loyal memory of the dearly departed.[17]

Long-lasting applause confirmed once more what Clemens Neisser had so appositely expressed.

# 7. Alzheimer's: The Career of a Disease

Emil Kraepelin coined the term *Alzheimer's disease* in 1910, when he used it for the first time on page 627 of the eighth, completely revised edition of his textbook. "The clinical interpretation of Alzheimer's disease is still unclear at the moment." The history of one of the best-known diseases begins with this sentence; it is a disease that even today is clouded with uncertainty.

At the beginning of the twentieth century, Kraepelin was one of the most highly regarded psychiatrists. His textbook was a must for every medical student and for all psychiatrists in private practice and in hospitals. Kraepelin's clinic in Nussbaumstrasse was one of the most recognized in Germany and accommodated most visiting doctors. With such a reputation, Kraepelin was entitled to call a disease by the name of one of his best and most loyal co-workers and thus to raise the name *Alzheimer* to an eponym.

In the mid- and late nineteenth century, many different things were named after the first person to discover, observe, or describe them. Some names caught on all by themselves, as did *diesel fuel* or the *otto motor* (internal combustion engine).

In Germany, X rays are known as Röntgen rays because Würzburg physicist Wilhelm Conrad Röntgen discovered them. Parkinson's disease is named for the first person to describe it, James P. Parkinson, and the now-widespread process of preserving food was soon named pasteurization after its inventor, Louis Pasteur. The most important award for scientific or artistic achievement is also an eponym: the Nobel prize is named after its founder, the inventor of dynamite, Alfred Nobel.

In the case of Alzheimer's disease, the naming of this form of illness was a coup for Kraepelin. His chief physician, Alzheimer, attained the chair of psychiatry in Breslau. This meant an unequivocal increase in prestige for his clinic; previously only Gaupp and Nissl had been appointed to the position of *Ordinarius*, or full professor.

That Alzheimer could outshine Eugen Bleuler—at that time already a very well-known figure—was considered a sensation among experts in the

218 ALZHEIMER'S: THE CAREER OF A DISEASE

psychiatric world. Alzheimer had also stood out against the psychiatric stronghold of Prague, where Arnold Pick was at the top. Kraepelin had also wanted to establish—in opposition to Sigmund Freud's burgeoning new theory of psychoanalysis—a clinical picture that unqualifiedly demonstrated that psychological symptoms could be traced back to changes in the brain, not, as Freud asserted, to traumas in early childhood.

Kraepelin did not think much of psychoanalysis: "What is known so far about this interpretive art makes it appear completely conceivable that psychoanalysis could simply never become common property; it is obviously more art than science." That is why it was satisfying for him to see the chair in Breslau in the hands of a biologically oriented psychiatrist such as Alzheimer as well as predecessors such as Wernicke and Bonhoeffer, and Kraepelin also strove to assert his influence in this direction by filling other chairs.

Alzheimer's reaction to the eponym was surprising; he was rather self-critical at first. "Thus the question arises whether these cases of disease, which I have considered as peculiar, still show characteristic features in clinical and histologic aspects that distinguish them from senile dementia or whether they must be assigned instead to senile dementia itself."[1] Alzheimer wrote this at the beginning of 1911 in "On Peculiar Cases of Illness of Later Age," an article he submitted to the *Zeitschrift für die Gesamte Neurologie und Psychiatrie*. In the same article he discussed a case that seemed appropriate "to increase awareness of the difficulties that the clinical evaluation of these cases presents us with": the case of day laborer Johann F., the second case Alzheimer described.

However, the name *Alzheimer's disease* was introduced into world medical literature during Alzheimer's lifetime. It was Dr. Gonzalo R. Lafora, a histopathologist from Madrid, working as a guest doctor in Washington, D.C. at the laboratory of the Government Hospital for the Insane, who gave the first account of an American with Alzheimer's disease. At that time German was still the international language of science, and his publication was in that language. It concerned fifty-eight-year-old William C.F. His symptoms had begun in 1906, the year Auguste D. died.

He presented with excitation, disconnected speech, and ideas of persecution; he asked for protection. Several weeks earlier he had proposed marriage to several nurses. Shortly after the beginning of the illness he became negligent and dirty, wet himself, and then smeared his face and body with urine. Once, in a state of excitation, he threw an iron bar at a nurse. He was disoriented. He did not know the names of any of the doctors and nurses, nor did he know where he was. Very often he forgot the way to his room.

The following dialogue is reminiscent of Alzheimer's own manner of interviewing his patients:

"What day is it today?"

"I don't know exactly, missus."

"What is the date?"

"I don't know that, miss, man, mister."

"What month is it? What year?"

"Right under this corner, Mr. Man."

"How long have you been in this hospital?"

"Right there, miss, is everything that I know, I'm telling you."

"What kind of a house is this?"

"I don't know, I know nothing, absolutely nothing, nothing, nothing, zero."

"Where is it?"

"Hell hell hell hell hell hell hell."

"Where are you from?"

"I already told you. I was in Lancaster; I don't know anything."

The patient then said spontaneously that he had heard a pretty woman speaking.

"What did she say to you?"

"I don't know, ma'am, neither, if I told you about it or should tell you about it; it is pretty, pretty, cute, cute."

The article also says, "Later the patient frequently ate his own excrement, was negligent, destroyed his clothes, sometimes walked aimlessly from one place to another, or spent the entire day in bed."

Lafora correctly diagnosed William C.F. with Alzheimer's disease. Alzheimer, then editor of the *Zeitschrift für die Gesamte Neurologie und Psychiatrie,* received the article on May 27, 1911, and immediately accepted it for publication.[2]

Nevertheless, when Alzheimer died in 1915, the disease named after him generally was not mentioned in the many remembrances of him. Even Max Lewandowsky, Alzheimer's co-editor at the *Zeitschrift für die Gesamte Neurologie und Psychiatrie,* did not mention it.

And what is more astonishing is that even Kraepelin did not mention Alzheimer's disease, although it was he who had introduced the concept to the medical world.

Nissl's contribution is still more astonishing; it does not mention Alzheimer's disease but remarks, "The histopathologist Alzheimer often is described as my student. I could honestly not be more proud of anything than of being named with the glorious title of his teacher."[3]

However, Alzheimer's son-in-law, Georg Stertz, knew exactly what was at stake: "There is just one group of illnesses that I would especially like to single out, because they bear Alzheimer's name. It concerns rare cases of an illness in presenility, appearing in the forties and quite rapidly leading to deepest stupor, which appears interesting from both a clinical and a research perspective because alongside the mental infirmity appear diagnostic, aphasic, and apraxic symptoms that border on purely psychological associative and focal signs."[4]

Walter Spielmeyer, Alzheimer's successor in Munich, wrote a forty-one-page obituary in which he expressly referred to Alzheimer's disease:

In 1906 Alzheimer described a remarkable process that he himself described as a peculiar, previously unknown disease, the most striking anatomic symptom of which was the deposit of strange substances in the cerebral cortex and the reorganization of fibrils into thick bundles and networks. He repeatedly returned to the material he had compiled in Frankfurt when he acquainted us with this peculiar disease of the cortex that we today follow Kraepelin in calling "Alzheimer's disease."[5]

Karl Kleist had been director of the University Psychiatric Clinic in Frankfurt since 1920. There, in the mid-1920s, he and a co-worker examined patient M.A. and immediately decided to make a teaching film. The film was described in the program of the *Medizinischen Filmwoche* (*Medical Film Weekly*):

Mrs. M.A. initially presented as a fearful and depressive clinical picture with memory deficits. A condition of extreme forgetfulness soon developed. This was soon accompanied by aphasia and disorders in linguistic comprehension and recognition. Finally, she can no longer carry out simple tasks, communication is impossible; her only spontaneous expressions are meaningless repetitions of sounds.

She falls into a stereotypic and iterative restless activity and spends the entire day fiddling with her bedding and pulls the pillowcases off the pillows. It looks in part as if she were washing, or dressing dolls, like a child; often no coherent action is recognizable, only individual partial actions such as plucking, putting things down and the like.[6]

The film, lost until now, may be the very first film ever about someone afflicted with Alzheimer's.

After 1919, Georg Stertz became chief physician in Munich; Kraepelin had brought him back to his own clinic after Alzheimer's death, after he had been deputy head of the Breslau clinic for two years.

Stertz took a position "On the Question of Alzheimer's Disease" in the *Allgemeinen Zeitschrift für Psychiatrie* (*General Journal of Psychiatry*) in 1921–1922. He could support his claims with the results of the examination of twenty-two cases from the Munich and Breslau clinics. His explanations point unequivocally to the future in that he, like Kraepelin, concluded "that Alzheimer's disease does not, as such, lead to death."[7]

Stertz said that Kraepelin was right in "recognizing presenile dementia as a distinct form of illness and in acknowledging the purposeful anatomic–clinical work of its discoverer, Alzheimer, by giving it his name, under which it later found widespread interest, without it being possible to say that the wealth of problems that reside therein have as yet been exhausted in any way."

In Würzburg in 1925 Dr. Ernst Grünthal, working at the Clinic for Psychiatric Illnesses, published an extensive work on Alzheimer's disease. Apparently Grünthal had taken fourteen brains with him from Munich to Würzburg. In Munich the patients had been "clinically observed with special attention, mostly over a long time, and uniformly diagnosed, for the most part by Kraepelin himself."

Grünthal came to a sensational conclusion: "At the moment, at least with our methods, a differential diagnosis between senile dementia and Alzheimer's disease cannot be made on the basis of histopathological images."[8]

222 ALZHEIMER'S: THE CAREER OF A DISEASE

A year later, Grünthal published another work on "Clinical–Anatomic Comparative Examinations of Senile Dementia." Patients under seventy years of age were not examined; in other words, no genuine cases of Alzheimer's disease were included. Again Grünthal came to an almost prophetic conclusion:

On a differential diagnosis in contrast to Alzheimer's disease one can say that the kind of histologic changes do not at present permit any distinction. Clinically, too, certain cases of senile dementia allow hardly any distinction from mild and moderate cases of Alzheimer's other than through age. However, an essential difference appears to me to be the often premature appearance of speech disorders, especially nominal aphasia, in Alzheimer's disease, which only rarely, even in severe cases, manifests in senile dementia.[9]

It is striking that the disease designation for young people with dementia was *Alzheimer's disease*; for the aged, in contrast, ugly names such as *Greisenblödsinn* ("old person's stupidity") and *Greisenschwachsinn* ("old person's imbecility") were used.

In 1932 Johannes Schottky wrote an extensive article that continued to use the designation *presenile stupor*. Of his nineteen cases, nine were Alzheimer's disease cases in the narrower sense. Eugenie D. belonged in this latter category. She was the patient for whom Schottky was the first to pursue the question of heritability:

In the dark that still lies over the actual causes of the processes of senile stupefaction, a more precise examination of its hereditary basis, even with negative results, can still contribute to its clarification.

In the case of Eugenie D., the father (case 8) fell ill at age fifty-six of a quite similar complaint to that of the daughter (case 12), who died of the illness. This case provided the earliest age of illness of the entire series (forty-three years old) and is remarkable in every respect. Both the father and the daughter have a strong sex drive. Striking is also the mother of the father (case 4), who died at seventy-two after she had been childish and unclean for six

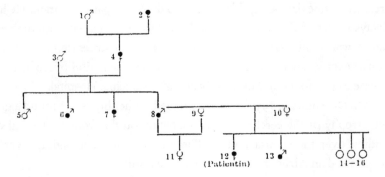

FIGURE 7.1 *Eugenie D.'s heredity chart*

years. It was probably a case of senile dementia; the grandmother
of the father also suffered from a mental illness.

Schottky thus found in Eugenie D. "an acquired stupor that ran
through four generations and appeared at ever younger years in the last
three generations; at very least in the cases of the father and daughter this
stupor bore strikingly similar traits."

The results of the additional neurologic examination in the case of Eugenie D. were remarkable: Several spinal taps show completely normal fluid. An encephalographic examination in which the cerebral ventricles are
filled with air was carried out in the X-ray unit of the Munich–Schwabing
Municipal Hospital and produced an interesting result:

A substantial filling stood out in the periphery, probably between
the individual gyri. In the side picture appeared, apart from the
ventricular filling, a substantial buildup of air in the front parts of
the skull. Also, over and also somewhat below the ventricular filling were irregular, band-shaped air elucidations. Especially given
the involvement of the forebrain, it therefore unquestionably appeared to be an indication of brain atrophy. Two days after the encephalography, by the way, a temporary clinical improvement
was noticeable.[10]

This diagnosis, the first X-ray results of the skull after filling the cerebral ventricles with air, is remarkable insofar as Alzheimer had always

dreamed of one day being able to see into the living patient's brain. He had always regretted that one could do little during the patient's lifetime and had to wait until death to investigate the internal structure of the brain. Consequently, the beginnings of the visual representation of Alzheimer's disease can be found in Munich–Swabing's Municipal Hospital.

On December 6, 1930, Eugenie D. died. In her brain was found a general atrophy of the cerebrum, predominantly on the frontal lobe and extending over the central region. The microscopic examination revealed plaques and an Alzheimerian disease of the fibrilla.

From August 22 to 25, 1936, the Society of German Neurologists and Psychiatrists met in Frankfurt for their second annual assembly. Doctor Pittrich and his superior, Karl Kleist, were very interested in iterative ergasiomania, a constant urge for activity, which he had often observed in demented patients, and he presented a remarkable lecture, which he illustrated with slides.[11] He presented a seventy-year-old patient whom he diagnosed as having Alzheimer's disease.

> The patient himself has mentally regressed in recent years. In the last three quarters of a year he has begun to give confused answers and cry a lot; he is unclean and can no longer find his way to the toilet. In the last four months before admission he could no longer make himself understood and struggled against being washed and fed.

A series of impressive slides followed. One saw the patient incessantly in activity, running his hands over his face, stroking his hair back, rubbing his hands against each other, running his hand along his thigh, and plucking the palm of his left hand with his right. These movements were repeated uniformly. Pittrich called this striking behavior "stereotypic iterative ergasiomania" and continued,

> The facial expression is thoroughly attentive; the attention appears to be turned to the individual activity in question. The face also participates in the restlessness, as the following slide shows:
>
> > The lower lip is turned forward, the upper lip is pulled in, the tongue shoved out, and the mouth drawn wide. He snaps at a finger brought to his mouth and sucks on it, a so-called snap-and-

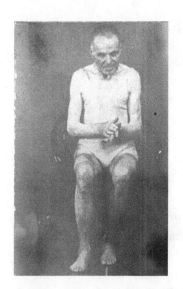
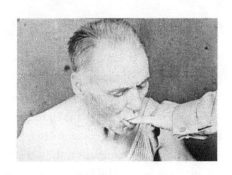
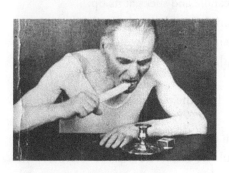
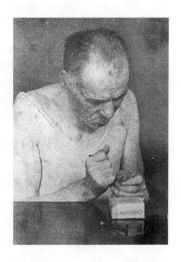
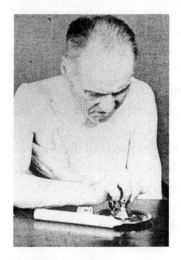
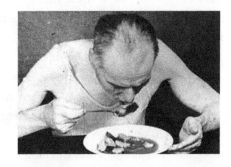

FIGURE 7.2 *Slides illustrating a lecture on a seventy-year-old patient with Alzheimer's disease (1936)*

suck reflex. A tamper, tobacco, and matches are laid by the patient on a table and a pipe put into his hands. He tries to take the pipe apart and then shoves the tamper and pipe together.

A candle is put in his right hand, and a candlestick and matches are placed on the table. He puts the candle on the table, makes screwing movements on the neck of the candlestick, takes several matches out of the box, places them in an orderly fashion next to each other between thumb and index finger, and touches them with the matchbox—not the striking surface, however, but rather the narrow side, and then pushes the matches toward his mouth like a fork, wipes with them on the table as if he wanted to pick something up, and then brings them up again to his oncoming mouth. Then he picks up the candle and sucks at its tip.

He uses a napkin ring to drink. He obviously does not recognize the objects, is blind to their significance, which we designate mind blindness [visual agnosia].

In conclusion Pittrich showed how the patient consumed a nutritious soup with great pleasure.

After the slides followed a film about the patient in which the patterns of movement and his disorders could be seen. The signs of "stereotypic iterative ergasiomania" were accepted by the participants as an impressive symptom of dementia. The seven and a half minute film has been preserved and, unless an earlier one is found, must be considered the world's first film documenting Alzheimer's disease. The microscopic investigations carried out by privatdozent Stadler in the clinic's histopathological laboratory showed typical results: Alzheimer-type changes in the fibrilla and numerous senile plaques. At autopsy the brain was extremely atrophied and weighed only 1100 grams.

What was remarkable in this case was that Pittrich used the diagnosis *Alzheimer's disease* for a seventy-year-old, that is, for a patient with senile dementia. He thus took a leap toward unifying the disease nomenclature.

In the years that followed little mention was made of Alzheimer's disease; only from the early 1960s can documents be found that show that the designation *Alzheimer's* was catching on at congresses.

In Berlin in December 1962 two patients presented clinically: one with Alzheimer's and the other with Pick's disease, an atrophy of forebrain.

Afterward, Elfriede Albert of Düsseldorf gave a remarkable lecture: "Senile Dementia and Alzheimer's: The Same Disease?"

In 1964 she published this lecture in full under the title "Senile Dementia and Alzheimer's Disease as Expressions of the Same Disease Event." The essay is dedicated to her teacher, Prof. Karl Kleist, and runs about fifty pages. In it, Albert sees no distinction in principle between the premature stupor of Alzheimer's disease and actual senile dementia: "Alzheimer himself had already decided against a distinction in principle between presenile stupor and senile dementia. All the same, a patient with Alzheimer's is expected to show a more abrupt course of disease."[12]

Albert introduced a new concept: "Alzheimerization." She thus designated a process by which the abrupt onset of Alzheimer's exacerbates an existing senile dementia. "Thus, for example, the patient Sch. had already suffered for three years from an insidious senile dementia, when under exogenous damage the process of a classic Alzheimer's disease developed."

From this medical case the author deduced that Alzheimer's disease could develop as an acute syndrome emerging from a senile dementia. Therefore, she argued, Alzheimer's must be a part of the same process, which becomes more acute and intense and therefore leads far more rapidly to severe brain defects. With the help of detailed analyses of patients' speech Albert discovered that the linguistic regression found in senile dementia and that found in Alzheimer's disease were fundamentally the same. She concluded that there was no distinction, either anatomically or clinically, between the two diseases.

It was not long before an international congress looked into the theme of dementia. A symposium, "Senile Dementia: Clinical and Therapeutic Aspects," was held from September 15 to 17, 1967, in Lausanne. The event was organized by analytically oriented physicians: Prof. C. Mueller and Dr. L. Ciompi from the University Psychiatric Clinic in Lausanne.

The participants, who included Elfriede Albert, came from throughout Europe. J. E. Meyer and H. Lauter, both from the University Psychiatric Clinic in Göttingen, set a milestone in the recognition of Alzheimer's disease. They spoke about clinical and classificatory conceptions of senile dementia, and Lauter summarized his results as follows: "In agreement with other physicians we regard senile dementia and Alzheimer's disease as a unit of illness that manifests at distinct ages. The term *Alzheimer's dementia* is therefore proposed."[13]

Shortly afterward, Albert spoke on the forms of illness in the demented, explained her concept of "Alzheimerization," and finally fused the concepts of presenile and senile dementia.[14] It was high time because in Europe and America, cases of this illness were accumulating.

However, many still believed that arteriosclerosis, or, as it was popularly called, "calcification of the arteries," was responsible for causing senile dementia. With advancing age, arteriosclerotic deposits in the vessels damage the arterial walls in all organs, but particularly in the brain.

It was also widely believed that certain groups of people, such as marathon runners, did not develop arteriosclerotic changes. Yet when postmortems were finally carried out on marathon runners, changes in the coronary blood vessels similar to those of nonrunners were found in several of them. The myth of the arteriosclerotic origin of senile dementia therefore could not be sustained.

In the 1960s a number of British pathologists examined the blood vessels of people who had died of dementia and compared them with the blood vessels of people who, at the time of death, had shown no signs of mental illness. They found approximately the same degree of arteriosclerotic change in those who had been demented and those who had not.[15]

Another team of pathologists repeated the work and examined more than one hundred brains; they also found that arteriosclerotic changes did not appear any more often in the brains of those with senile dementia.

In 1966 the breakthrough finally came when Bernard E. Tomlinson, Gary Blessed, and Martin Roth made public their epoch-making work. They had clinically investigated fifty demented patients and, after their deaths, performed autopsies on them and histopathologically analyzed their brains. The authors then compared their results with those of elderly controls who did not suffer from dementia—healthy people—and came to a result that no one had expected: More than half of the demented people showed pathological results that indicated Alzheimer's disease.[16]

However, myths usually live to a ripe old age: Only in 1974 was an official refutation of "calcification theory" announced. Vladimir C. Hachinski declared succinctly, "The use of the concept 'calcification of the arteries of the brain' to describe mental decline in the aged probably is the most common misdiagnosis in medicine."[17]

In this way Alzheimer's disease became the most frequently attributed cause of the mental decline of older people who had previously been labeled with *Greisenblödsinn* and later with senile dementia.

Alzheimer's disease would have remained rare and ultimately insignificant if not for something that had not previously occurred in human history: the gradual increase of the mean life expectancy of people living in highly industrialized countries.

The improvement of hygienic and social conditions, in conjunction with the successes of modern medicine in preventing and controlling epidemics and improving nutrition, had all contributed to the fact that the general life expectancy of people in Europe and America had doubled in the last 300 years. Whereas at the time of the French Revolution the average life expectancy was about thirty years, it now lies, apart from the effects of war, at seventy to eighty years in industrialized nations, and this figure is still rising.

Around sixty years ago Danish writer Ellen Key called the twentieth century the "century of the child." By the century's end it had become one of older people, even of the elderly. In 1920 people over age sixty made up 5 percent of the population; today the figure stands at 20 to 25 percent. In 1900 the mean life expectancy in Germany was around forty-seven years for men and fifty years for women. Today this expectancy is around seventy-two years for men and seventy-eight years for women.

And because women have a higher life expectancy than men, among people over sixty years women clearly outnumber men. This is particularly noticeable in the highest age groups such as 100-year-olds.

The cover story of the *Ärtzeblatt* (*Doctor's Paper*) of February 27, 1998, "The Early Death of the Stronger Sex," reports, "In Germany women live on average more than six years longer than men. The differences in states of health become clear only with age; however, the causes lie much further back. Among other things, the fulfillment of typical masculine roles is bound up with high risks to health."[18]

Social support for the older generation is regarded as increasingly necessary, but it is men in particular who could profit most from it because traditional male social relations and networks are mostly activity- and work-oriented and clearly do more harm to health than the predominantly emotional, long-term social relationships of women.

The higher life expectancy of women has a cause: In the autopsies of ninety-year-old women one finds on average six "categories of illness"

(*Krankheitseinheiten*) or defects, whereas in men of the same age on average eight to nine impairments can be diagnosed. Interestingly, this fact holds true for all mammals.

So why do people dream of an ever longer life? The prospects certainly are not all pleasant. If we really want to live for 100 years, then the risk of falling ill with Alzheimer's stands at 50 percent. In the United States the disease is the fourth most common cause of death; more than 100,000 people die of it annually. In the retirement homes of all highly industrialized lands, more than half of all of the occupants suffer from a dementia.

A Brothers Grimm tale of the nineteenth century can be read as a warning:

When God had created the world and wanted to choose the lifespans of all of the creatures, the donkey came to him and asked, "Lord, how long will I live?" "Thirty years," answered God. "Does that suit you?" "Oh Lord," replied the donkey, "that is a long time. Consider my arduous existence: From morning until night I must bear heavy burdens, carry sacks of corn to the mill, so that others may eat bread, and I am encouraged and refreshed by nothing but kicks and blows! Waive for me a part of this long time." God had mercy and gave him eighteen years.

The donkey went away consoled, and the dog appeared. "How long do you want to live?" said God to the dog. "For the donkey thirty years are too many, but you will be satisfied with that." "Lord," answered the dog, "is that your will? Consider how much I have to run; my feet will not hold out; and when I no longer have voice enough to bark nor teeth enough to bite, what is left for me but to run from one corner to another and to snarl?" God saw that the dog was right and granted him twelve years.

Then came the monkey. "You must want to live for thirty years," said the Lord to him. "You do not need to work like the donkey and the dog, and you are always in good spirits." "Oh Lord," he answered, "it looks that way, but it isn't so. When it rains millet seeds, I don't have a spoon. I am always supposed to pull amusing pranks, make funny faces, so that the people laugh, but when they pass me an apple and I bite into it, it's sour. How often is sadness hidden behind all the fun! Thirty years—I couldn't cope." God was merciful and gave him ten years.

Finally man appeared. He was joyful, healthy, and fresh, and asked God to determine his time. "Thirty years shall you live," spoke the Lord. "Is that enough for you?" "What a short time!" cried the man. "When I have built my house, and a fire burns in my own stove, when I have planted trees that blossom and bear fruits, and I intend to enjoy my life, then I should die? Oh, Lord, extend my time!" "I will add on for you the eighteen years of the donkey," said God. "That is not enough," replied the man. "You shall also have the twelve years of the dog." "Still not enough!" "Well now," said God, "I will give you the ten years of the monkey, but you will not get any more." The man went away but was not satisfied.

So man lives seventy years. The first thirty are his human years, and they pass quickly; during them he is healthy and cheerful, works with enthusiasm, and enjoys his existence. After that follow the eighteen years of the donkey, in which one burden after another is laid upon him: He has to carry the corn that nourishes others, and kicks and blows are the wages of his loyal service. Then come the twelve years of the dog, in which he lies in the corners, snarls, and no longer has teeth to bite with. And when this time is over, the ten years of the monkey bring a conclusion. Then the man is idiotic and foolish, does silly things, and becomes a laughingstock to children.

Apart from the public ridicule to which the afflicted herself was initially exposed, Alzheimer's disease increasingly challenged the daughter of a world-famous woman who had developed Alzheimer's disease by the time she was forty-two years old. In 1960 the magazine *Film und Frau* (*Film and Woman*) had already remarked, "Rita Hayworth radiates glamour but has to expend all of her energy to ignite it."

No one can say for sure whether these were the first signs of Alzheimer's disease. Strange changes gradually took place in Rita Hayworth. She became scared to go into remote corners of her home by herself and began to cry out spontaneously or blindly and to accuse others unfairly.

FIGURE 7.3  *Rita Hayworth in* Gilda *(1946)*

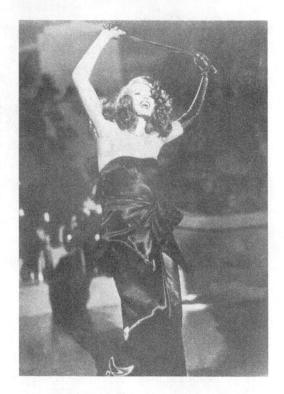

Soon afterward she repeatedly forgot what she had to say, and films had to be shot line by line.

In the early years Fred Astaire, her partner in many world-famous films, had been deeply impressed by how quickly she had learned. When he showed her new steps before lunch, after lunch she had mastered them perfectly: "She must have practiced the number in her head during the meal," he said, astonished. "But now nothing stuck anymore."

In 1977 she embarked on a cure for alcoholism. She presented the horrifying image of a lonely drinker who threw empty gin bottles over the hedge at her neighbor, movie star Glenn Ford. When she wandered through the streets of Beverly Hills, unkempt and absent-minded, she carried a note in her purse on which her address was written. She was classified as an alcoholic, but no one realized that she drank only out of despair over her breakdown.

Her daughter Yasmin, her child from her third marriage, with Prince Ali Khan, tried to make clear to her who she was. She put her mother in front of the mirror and said, pointing to the mirror image, "See, that's you, Rita Hayworth!" But her mother just stared at her red hair, the only thing that had not lost its gleam.

In 1981 the doctors diagnosed Alzheimer's disease, and Yasmin had to assume guardianship. Rita Hayworth needed 'round-the-clock care from nurses and her daughter. The once captivatingly beautiful actress and dancer slept twelve hours a day; the rest she spent staring dully.

In 1984, at age sixty-four, she was in the last stages of Alzheimer's disease. The "Love Goddess," who fell prey at the end of her life to a form of living decay, could hardly speak. If she said anything at all, it was often, "He does it like this" or "He showed me how I should do it." Perhaps they were instructions from actor and director Orson Welles, her fourth husband, that had engraved themselves in her long-term memory.

On May 14, 1987, the actress died in her New York apartment, legally incapacitated, paralyzed, and deranged. The physicians had in the meantime freed her from the suspicion of alcoholism: It was not alcohol but rather the pernicious brain disease that had afflicted her mind and body. Yasmin released the doctors from their confidentiality obligations, ensuring that her famous mother would make the term *Alzheimer's disease* known throughout the world.

The last years of Rita Hayworth's life were very similar to those of Auguste D., whom Alois Alzheimer had examined for the first time in 1901 in the Municipal Mental Asylum in Frankfurt. Both were cases of classic Alzheimer's, Alzheimer's in the narrower sense, which is distinguished as a brain disease that appears as the result of an as yet unknown cause in the fifth or sixth decade of life and is bound up with an atrophy of the cerebral cortex.[19]

Another internationally known person went still further and himself admitted his illness: In November 1994 former U.S. president Ronald Reagan said farewell to the public in a letter:

> I have recently been told that I am one of millions of Americans with Alzheimer's disease. Nancy and I had to decide whether we would keep this matter to ourselves as private citizens or would make it known. We had the feeling that it was important to announce this message publicly.[20]

FIGURE 7.4 *Ronald Reagan*

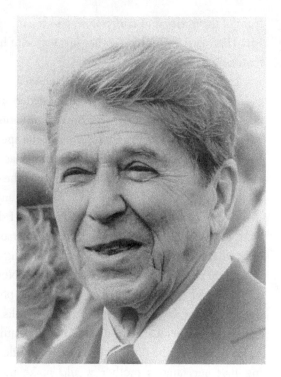

Things have gotten very dark around Reagan, now ninety-one years old. He can barely recall his eight-year presidency. Politics no longer interests him. He receives his visitors politely, but he does not know who they are. His vocabulary diminishes more and more.

Reagan's frank letter on the painful experience of his mental decline had the intended effect: The term *Alzheimer's disease* was used more often. According to an estimate by Robert Katzman in a 1976 article in *Archives of Neurology*, Alzheimer's disease is the fourth most common cause of death in the United States, yet in none of the death statistics do the terms *Alzheimer's*, *senile dementia*, or *senility* appear. Katzman calls for the use of the disease term *Alzheimer's* in place of *senile dementia* and for a repudiation of the age distinction.[21]

Katzman's appeal had noticeable consequences in the United States but fewer in Europe. As a result of the clear disease definition and in view of the enormous number of patients afflicted, in 1967 a U.S. government conference led to the establishment of the National Institute of Aging within the National Institutes of Health. From there, and from many other

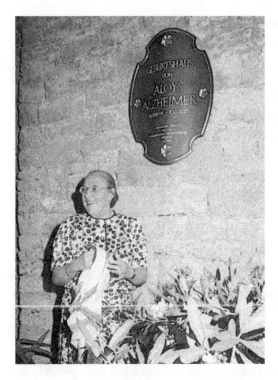

FIGURE 7.5
*In 1989 Alzheimer's grand-daughter Hildegard Koeppen unveiled a memorial plaque at the birth house in Marktbreit.*

sources, flowed the means for inquiry into age-related illnesses, especially Alzheimer's disease.

Since prominent people such as Rita Hayworth and Ronald Reagan have admitted that they have the disease, substantial funds have been made available, and many research centers on Alzheimer's disease have been founded.

In June 1989 an international symposium on the 125th birthday of Alois Alzheimer took place in Würzburg and Marktbreit, his birthplace. The organizers were the University Psychiatric Clinics in Würzburg and Munich and the Institute for Pathobiochemistry of the University of Heidelberg.

The news magazine *Der Spiegel* held Alzheimer's 125th birthday to be so important that they devoted a cover story to him.[22] At the house where Alzheimer was born, his granddaughter Hildegard Koeppen unveiled a memorial plaque. In 1995 Alzheimer's birthplace was donated to the public on the eightieth anniversary of his death as a conference center and memorial site.

However, in the mid-1980s doubts arose about the diagnosis of Auguste D. Many began to suspect that she actually had arteriosclerosis or perhaps a rare neurologic disease. But Alois Alzheimer was vindicated, as noted in the science section of the *Frankfurter Allgemeine Zeitung* in April 1998:

> Psychiatrist Alois Alzheimer, active in Frankfurt am Main, was not mistaken in his initial diagnosis of the disease that was named after him. The patient he examined, Auguste D., did actually suffer from Alzheimer's dementia. . . . Researchers in Martinsried only recently stumbled across the long-missing brain slide preparations. They saw the characteristic neurofibrillary bundles and amyloid plaques. They did not find signs of a vascular-conditioned dementia.

Toward the end of the twentieth century, the concepts of presenile and senile dementia have become fused, with the effect that the eponym *Alzheimer's disease* has been used for all dementias. Sometimes the term is used in a way that turns on its head the classic conception of Alzheimer's, which sets in early, as when a headline in the *Hamburger Abendblatt* of February 25, 1998, asked, "Alzheimer's in Younger Years?" and continued, "Alzheimer's disease is of course called senile dementia but may possibly already begin in younger years."

Alois Alzheimer's name has entered the vernacular like no other physician's. And although *Alzheimer* is sometimes shortened to *Alzi* and often used in a joking way—"Greetings from Alzheimer!"—these words will stick in the throat of anyone who has had to care, even for a short time, for a person who suffers from this dreadful disease, which can strike any person, regardless of background or lifestyle.

There is no cure for this destructive illness, despite research being conducted throughout the world. Drugs that stem the disease, improve symptoms, and substantially delay its course are available and are a great help for the afflicted.

Brain training is well on its way to becoming a popular sport. Patients with Alzheimer's disease, affected relatives, and healthy people alike benefit from the training. More and more people are adopting methods that are simple, yet all the more effective for that, and thus are increasing the efficiency of their brains.

The use of electronic devices, reports on which appeared in 1998, can help protect the sick from themselves: "Mildly confused occupants of the

Meander Nursing Home in Veendam can now no longer escape unnoticed. Computer chips have been installed in the shoes of the thirty seniors, most of whom suffer from Alzheimer's. The director of the home says, 'In the elevators and outside doors, electronic detectors give off a peep signal as soon as someone with the specially prepared shoes comes into the vicinity.' Result: The doors close automatically."[23]

The greatest burden weighs on the shoulders of the caretakers, usually next of kin, who sacrifice themselves in an almost superhuman fashion for the sick. They can only watch as their loved ones decline more and more and no longer even know the answer to the simple question posed by the doctor in attendance: "What is your name?"

## Family Tree

*Alzheimer's great-grand parents*
Michael Johann Alzheimer    ∞    Margarethe Gunther
b. 1757                              b. 1768

*Alzheimer's grand parents*
Johann Alzheimer    ∞    Crescentia Bachmann
1797–1882                             b. 1768

*First marriage of Eduard Alzheimer*
Eduard Alzheimer    ∞    Eva Maria Sabina Busch
1830–1891                           1840–1882

Karl Eduard Sebastian
1862–1924

*Second marriage of Eduard Alzheimer*
Eduard Alzheimer    ∞    Barbara Theresia Busch
1830–1891                           1840–1882

| Alois | Johanna | Eduard | Alexander | Elisabeth | Alfred |
|-------|---------|--------|-----------|-----------|--------|
| 1864–1915 | 1865–1920 | 1867–1848 | 1870–1942 | 1872–1968 | 1875–1949 |

*Third marriage of Eduard Alzheimer*
Eduard Alzheimer    ∞    Martha Katharina Maria Geiger
1863–1891

Eugenia
1884–1950

Alois Alzheimer    ∞    Cecil b. Wallerstein,
                                  widowed Geisenheimer
June 14, 1864–December 19, 1915    July 6, 1860–February 28, 1901

| Gertrud, married name Stertz | Hans Eduard | Maria, married name Finsterwalder |
|------------------------------|-------------|-----------------------------------|
| 1895–1980 | 1896–1981 | 1900–1977 |
| Hildegard Koeppan Gabriele Hager | Ilse Lieblein Kerin Weise | Barbara Lipper Rupert Finsterwalder |

# Chronology

June 14, 1864 Alois Alzheimer is born in the early morning

1870–1874 Attends elementary school in Marktbreit

1874–1878 Moves to Aschaffenburg and enters Royal Humanistic *Gymnasium*

1884–1888 Studies medicine

1887 Writes thesis "On the Earwax Glands"

1888 Completes state examinations and earns certification with the grade "very good"

Works at Albert von Kölliker's histologic laboratory

Works as travel companion to a mentally ill woman

Works as an intern at the Municipal Asylum for the Insane and Epileptic in Frankfurt under Emil Sioli

1892 Publishes "On a Case of Progressive Spinal Muscle Atrophy"

1895 Marries Cecilie Simonette Nathalie Geisenheimer, née Wallerstein; daughter Gertrud is born

Publishes "Paralysis Progressiva in Juveniles"

Is promoted to chief physician at the Frankfurt Asylum for the Insane and Epileptic

1896 Son, Hans, is born

1900 Daughter Maria is born

1901 Wife, Cecilie, dies

Fifty-one-year-old Auguste D. is admitted with symptoms of a dementia in November

1902 Moves to Heidelberg to work with Emil Kraepelin as scientific assistant

1903 Moves with Kraepelin to the psychiatric clinic in Munich

Directs the brain anatomy laboratory

1904 Submits *Habilitation* thesis, "Histologic Studies on the Differential Diagnosis of General Paresis"

1906 Presents "On a Peculiar Disease of the Cerebral Cortex," the first description of a presenile dementia, later named *Alzheimer's disease* at Kraepelin's suggestion

1910 First mention of the designation *Alzheimer's disease* appears in Kraepelin's psychiatry textbook

1912 Accepts full professorship of psychiatry at the Psychiatric Clinic of the Silesian Friedrich-Wilhelm University in Breslau

1913 Stays at health spa in Wiesbaden

1915 Dies of kidney failure on December 19

Funeral is held at the main cemetery in Frankfurt on December 23

# Notes

## 1. The Auguste D. File

1. Auguste D. File, 1901–1906. Clinic of the Johann-Wolfgang-Goethe University at Frankfurt am Main, Department of Psychiatry and Psychotherapy I, partly published in K. Maurer, S. Volk, and H. Gerbaldo, "Auguste D. and Alzheimer's Disease," in *Lancet* 349 (1997): 1546–1549.

2. Trans. note: In German, Alzheimer asks whether she hears *Stimmen*, and Auguste D. responds that she hears *Summen*.

## 2. Alois Alzheimer's Ancestry, Childhood, and Youth

1. K. Maurer, "Anmerkungen zum Geburtshaus, zur Person und zum Todestag von Alois Alzheimer," Lecture at the Symposium for the 80th anniversary of Alois Alzheimer's death and the opening of the birth house as a museum and conference center, Marktbreit, December 19, 1995 (unpublished).

2. O. Hansmann and J. Schirmer, *Marienwallfahrtsort Rengersbrunn* (Bad Soden, no date).

3. M. Goes, "Alois Alzheimer und die nach ihm benannte Krankheit," *Mitteilungen aus dem Stadt- und Stiftsarchiv Aschaffenburg* 3(2, September 1990): 77–83.

4. Gemeinde Biebergemünd anlässlich der 1000-Jahr-Feier, ed., *1000 Jahre Kassel und Wirtheim* (Gelnhausen, no date).

5. *Fürstlich Schwarzenberg'sches Wochenblatt*, June 24, 1862, No. 25.

6. R. Plochmann, *Urkundliche Geschichte der Stadt Marktbreit in Unterfranken* (Erlangen 1864).

7. This and the following documentary reports on Eduard Alzheimer and his family are from the Marktbreit Town Archive (unpublished).

8. Register of St. Ludwig's Parish, Marktbreit, now Episcopal Archive, Würzburg, Fol. I, p. 101.

9. See note 1.

## 3. Student of Medicine

1. J. Conolly, *The Treatment of the Insane Without Mechanical Restraint* (London 1856, reprinted 1973).

2. University Archive of the Humboldt University at Berlin, Leaving Certificate of Alois Alzheimer of March 11, 1884, Archive No. 714.

3. H. Fromm, "Alois Alzheimer: Ein übersehener bedeutender Corpsstudent," *Beiträge zur Geschichte des Corps Franconia zu Würzburg* 101 (1988): 1–18.

4. University Archive of the Julius-Maximilian University Würzburg, Registration Lists, Alois Alzheimer, for the Winter Semester 1884–85.

5. Frankfurt City Archive, Files of the Magistrate, Information Files Concerning the Frankfurt Municipal Mental Asylum, 1888, 230 II, Q 62 b.

6. Meeting of the Alzheimer Grandchildren on January 6, 1998 (Participants: Barbara Lippert, Ilse Lieblein, Hildegard Koeppen, Dr. Rupert Finsterwalder, and Karin Weiss), minutes taken by R. Finsterwalder (unpublished).

7. University Archive of the Eberhard-Karls University Tübingen, Alois Alzheimer Personnel Files 5/32.

8. M. Weiss, *Tausend Semester Tübingen* (Tübingen 1991).

9. A. Alzheimer, "Über die Ohrschmalzdrüsen," Inaugural Dissertation, Würzburg 1888.

10. University Archive of the Ludwig-Maximilian University Munich, Alois Alzheimer Personnel Files, E II N, 1888.

*4. From Würzburg to Frankfurt*

1. H. Hoffmann, *Beobachtungen und Erfahrungen über Seelenstörungen und Epilepsie* (Frankfurt am Main, 1859).

2. W. Enzensberger, "Der Struwwelpeter-Hoffmann," *Symbiose* 4 (1990): 27–31.

3. G. Groddeck, in G. H. Herzog, M. Herzog-Hoinkins, and H. Siefert, eds., *Heinrich Hoffmann, Leben und Werk in Texten und Bildern* (Frankfurt 1995).

4. Heinrich Hoffmann, *Lebenserinnerungen* (Frankfurt 1985).

5. Documentation for the advertisement for the position and A. Alzheimer's application in Frankfurt City Archive, File of the Municipal Authorities, Files for the Frankfurt Municipal Mental Asylum, 1888, 230 II–V.

6. H. Siefert, "Heinrich Hoffmann (1809–1894)" *Hessisches Ärtzeblatt* 5 (1988): 281–283.

7. See note 4.

8. Brigitte Leuchtweis-Gerlach, "Emil Sioli, der geistige Vater des Waldkrankenhauses Köppern," *Suleburc Chronik. Schriften zur Geschichte der Stadt Friedrichsdorf* 6 (1995): 3–18.

9. A. Alzheimer, "25 Jahre Psychiatrie," *Archiv für Psychiatrie und Nervenkrankheiten* 52 (1913): 853–866.

10. Emil Sioli, *Bericht über die Anstalt für Irre und Epileptische in Frankfurt am Main 1889* (Frankfurt 1889).

11. H. Spatz, "Franz Nissl," in W. Scholz, ed., *50 Jahre Neuropathologie in Deutschland* (Stuttgart 1961), pp. 43–66.

12. See note 9.

13. See note 10.

14. E. Kraepelin, "Die Heidelberger Wachabteilung für unruhige Kranke," *Allgemeine Zeitschrift für Psychiatrie* 59 (1902): 133–136.

15. A. Alzheimer, "Über einen Fall von spinaler progressiver Muskelatrophie und hinzutretender Erkrankung bulbärer Kerne und der Rinde," *Archiv für Psychiatrie und Nervenkrankheiten* 23 (1892): 459–485.

16. W. Krüke, "Carl Weigert," W. Scholz, ed., *50 Jahre Neuropathologie in Deutschland* (Stuttgart 1961): 5–18.

17. W. Krüke, "Ludwig Edinger," W. Scholz, ed., *50 Jahre Neuropathologie in Deutschland* (Stuttgart 1961): 21–32.

18. See note 9.

19. See note 9.

20. See note 10.

21. Documented in "Session Proceedings of the Conference of the Southwest German Psychiatrists in Karlsruhe, November 2–4, 1892," in *Neurologisches Zentralblatt* (1893).

22. See note 15.

23. E. Kraepelin, *Lebenserinnerungen*, H. Hippius, H. Peters, and H. Ploog, eds. (Berlin 1983), p. 76.

24. Published in A. Alzheimer, "Die arteriosklerotische Atrophie des Gehirns," *Allgemeine Zeitschrift für Psychiatrie und Psychisch-Gerichtliche Medizin* 51 (1895): 809–812.

25. Documented in "Annual Meeting of the Association of German Psychiatrists in Dresden on September 21 and 22, 1894," *Allgemeine Zeitschrift für Psychiatrie und Psychisch-Gerichtliche Medizin* 51 (1894): 809–812.

26. A. Alzheimer, "Die Paralysis progressiva der Entwicklungsjahre," *Neurologisches Zentralblatt* 13 (1894): 732.

27. A. Alzheimer, "Die Frühform der progressiven Paralyse," *Allgemeine Zeitschrift für Psychiatrische und Psychisch-Gerichtliche Medizin* 52 (1896): 533–594.

28. A. Alzheimer, "Ein geborener Verbrecher," *Archiv der Psychiatrie und Nervenkrankheiten* 28 (1896): 327–353.

29. C. Lombroso, *L'uomo delinquente* (Rome/Turin/Florence 1884).

30. H. Spatz, "Franz Nissl," in W. Scholz, ed., *50 Jahre Neuropathologie in Deutschland* (Stuttgart 1961), pp. 43–66.

31. A. Alzheimer, "Über die durch Druck auf den Augenapfel hervorgerufenen Visionen," *Zentralblatt für Nervenheilkunde und Psychiatrie* 18 (1895): 473–478.

32. A. Alzheimer, "Beiträge zur pathologischen Anatomie der Hirnrinde und zur anatomischen Grundlage einiger Psychosen," *Monatsschrift für Psychiatrie und Neurologie* 2 (1897): 82–120.

33. A. Alzheimer, "Beiträge zur pathologischen Anatomie der Epilepsie," *Monatsschrift für Psychiatrie und Neurologie* 4 (1898): 345–369.

34. A. Alzheimer, "Neuere Arbeiten über die Dementia senilis," *Monatsschrift für Psychiatrie und Neurologie* 3 (1898): 101–115.

35. Emil Sioli, *Bericht über die Anstalt für Irre und Epileptische in Frankfurt am Main 1899* (Frankfurt 1899).

36. Meeting of the Alzheimer grandchildren on January 6, 1998. Participants: Barbara Lippert, Ilse Lieblein, Hildegard Koeppen, Dr. Rupert Finsterwalder, and Karin Weiss, minutes taken by R. Finsterwalder (unpublished).

37. Franz Nissl, "Kleinere Mitteilungen zum Andenken an Alois Alzheimer," *Allgemeine Zeitschrift für Psychiatrie und Psychisch-Gerichtliche Medizin* 73 (1916): 96–107.

38. See note 11.

39. See note 38.

40. Documentation of the announcement of the position and A. Alzheimer's application in Frankfurt City Archive, Files of the Municipal Authorities, Files on the Frankfurt Municipal Insane Asylum, 1888, 230 III Q 16–28.

41. See note 37.

42. Emil Sioli, *Bericht über die Anstalt für Irre und Epileptische in Frankfurt am Main 1901* (Frankfurt 1901).

43. See note 8.

44. E. L. Hofmann, "Die ehemalige Trinkerheilstätte auf dem Burgberg bei Bieber," *Gemeinde Biebergemünd* (no year): 153–155.

## 5. To Munich via Heidelberg

1. E. Kraepelin, *Lebenserinnerungen*, ed. H. Hippius, H. Peters, and H. Ploog (Berlin 1983), p. 121.

2. H. Spatz, "Franz Nissl," in W. Scholz, ed. *50 Jahre Neuropathologie in Deutschland* (Stuttgart 1961), pp. 43–66.

3. "Über die Wachabteilungen der Heidelberger Irrenklinik," *Allgemeine Zeitschrift für Psychiatrie* 51 (1895): 1–21.

4. See note 1, p. 125.

5. Frankfurt City Archive, Personnel Files, Alois Alzheimer, 1903.

6. H. Kerschensteiner, "Geschichte der Münchner Krankenanstalten," in J. Bauer, ed., *Festschrift zum 100 jährigen Bestehen des Städtischen Krankenhauses links der Isar 1812–1913* (Munich 1913).

7. H. Hippius, ed., "Die Psychiatrische Klinik der Ludwig-Maximilians-Universität München," *Dokumente zur Baugeschichte* (München 1991).

8. See note 2.

9. H. Littmann, "Grundrissanlage und Aufbau," quoted in H. Hippius, ed., p. 52.

10. Bavarian Capital City Archive, Cultural Ministerial Files on the University of Munich, MK 11250.

11. German Volkskalendar for city and country for the year 1909, Odessa 1908.

12. See note 1, p. 133.

13. *Münchner Neueste Nachrichten* of November 7, 1904, No. 921.

14. See note 1, p. 135.

15. Documented in University Archive of the Ludwig-Maximilian University Munich, Personnel Files of Alois Alzheimer, E II N, 1904.

16. A. Alzheimer, *Histologische Studien zu Differentialdiagnose der progressiven Paralyse* (Jena 1904).

17. E. Kraepelin, *Psychiatrie. Ein Lehrbuch für Studierende und Ärzte*, 7th ed. (Leipzig 1907).

18. O. Bumke, *Lehrbuch der Geisteskrankheiten*, 3rd ed. (Munich 1917).

19. J. E. Meyer, "Alois Alzheimer," in W. Scholz, ed., *50 Jahre Neuropathologie in Deutschland* (Stuttgart 1961), pp. 67–78.

20. G. Macchi, C. Brahe, M. Pomponi, A. Alzheimer, and G. Perusini, "Should Man Divide What Fate United?," *European Journal of Neurology* 4 (1997): 210–213.

21. R. Gaupp, "Alois Alzheimer," *Münchner Medizinische Wochenschrift* 63 (1916): 195–196.

22. See note 19.

23. See note 1, p. 171.

24. See note 1, p. 149.

25. See note 10, MK 11255.

26. Published in A. Alzheimer, *"Delirium alcoholicum Magnans,"* *Zentralblatt für Nervenheilkunde und Psychiatrie* 27 (1904): 437–441.

27. T. Ziehen, *Psychiatrie für Ärzte und Studierende* (Berlin 1894).

28. A. Alzheimer, "Einiges über die anatomischen Grundlagen der Idiotie," *Zentralblatt für Nervenheilkunde und Psychiatrie* 27 (1904): 497–505.

29. A. Alzheimer, "Einige Methoden zur Fixierung der Cerebrospinalflüssigkeit," *Zentralblatt für Nervenheilkunde und Psychiatrie* 30 (1907): 449–451.

30. Published in A. Alzheimer, "Die Gruppierung der Epilepsie," *Allgemeine Zeitschrift für Psychiatrie und Psychisch-Gerichtliche Medizin* 64 (1907): 418–421.

31. Published in A. Alzheimer, "Haben wir bei den verschiedenen Geisteskrankheiten mit anatomischen Befund einen histologisch annähernd gleiden Krankheitsprozess, voranzuselzen?," *Neurologisches Zentralblatt* 24 (1805): 680–682.

32. Published in A. Hoche, "Kritisches zur psychischen Formenlehre," *Allgemeine Zeitschrift für Psychiatrie und Psychisch-Gerichtliche Medizin* 63 (1906): 559–563.

33. Published in E. Kraepelin and J. Lange, *Psychiatrie*, 9th ed. (Leipzig 1927).

34. See note 21.

35. E. Kraepelin, "Lebensschicksale deutscher Forscher," *Münchner Medizinische Wochenschrift* 3 (1920): 75–78.

36. "Über die Indikationen für eine künstliche Schwangerunterbrechung bei Geisteskranken," *Münchner Medizinische Wochenschrift* 54 (1907): 1617–1621.

37. K. Binding and A. Hoche, *Die Freigabe der Vernichtung lebensunwerten Lebens: ihr Massund ihre Form* (Leipzig 1922).

38. A. Alzheimer, "Beiträge zur Kenntnis der pathologischen Neuroglia und ihren Beziehungen in den Abbauvorgängen im Nervengewebe," F. Nissl and A. Alzheimer, *Histologische und histopathologische Arbeiten über die Grosshirnrinde* (Leipzig 1911).

39. A. Alzheimer, "Ist die Einrichtung einer psychiatrischen Abteilung im Reichsgesundheitsamt erstrebenswert?," *Zeitschrift für die Gesamte Neurologie und Psychiatrie* 6 (1911): 242–246.

40. Documented in *Zentralblatt für Nervenheilkunde und Psychiatrie* (1907): 177–179.

41. Published in A. Alzheimer, "Über eine eigenartige Erkrankung der Hirnrinde," *Allgemeine Zeitschrift für Psychiatrie und Psychisch-Gerichtliche Medizin* 64 (1907): 146–148.

42. G. Aschaffenburg, "Die Beziehungen des sexuellen Lebens zur Entstehung von Nerven- und Geisteskrankheiten," *Münchner Medizinische Wochenschrift* 37 (1906).

43. *Tübinger Chronik*, November 5, 1906.

44. G. Perusini, "Über klinische und histopathologische eigenartige psychische Erkrankungen des späteren Lebensalters," in F. Nissl and A. Alzheimer, eds., *Histopathologische Arbeiten über die Grosshirnrinde unter besonderer Berüksichtigung der pathologischen Anatomie der Geisteskrankheiten*, Vol. 3 (Leipzig 1911): 297–351.

45. See note 1, p. 172.

46. E. Kraepelin, *Psychiatrie. Ein Lehrbuch für Studierende und Aertze* (Leipzig, Vol. 1, 1909; Vol. 2, 1910).

47. A. Alzheimer, "Über eigenartige Krankheitsfalle des späteren Alters," *Zeitschrift für die Gesamte Neurologie und Psychiatrie* 4 (1911): 356–385.

48. See note 47, pp. 624–628.

49. *Frankfurter Rundschau* June 4, 1997, No. 126/23.

50. See note 10, MK 11245.

51. E. Kraepelin, "Lebensschicksale deutscher Forscher," *Münchner Medizinische Wochenschrift* 3 (1920): 75–78.

52. A. Alzheimer, "Die diagnostischen Schwierigkeiten in der Psychiatrie," *Zeitschrift für die Gesamte Neurologie und Psychiatrie* 1 (1910): 1–19.

53. A. Alzheimer, "Über Degeneration und Regeneration an der peripheren Nervenfaser," *Zeitschrift für die Gesamte Neurologie und Psychiatrie* 1 (1910): 654–655.

54. J. E. Meyer, "Alois Alzheimer," in K. Kolle, ed., *Gross Nervenärzte*, Vol. 2 (Stuttgart 1964).

55. Franz Nissl, "Kleinere Mittelungen zum Andenken an Alois Alzheimer," *Allgemeine Zeitschrift für Psychiatrie und Psychisch-Gerichtliche Medizin* 73 (1916): 96–107.

56. See note 21.

57. See note 15.

58. See note 1, p. 171.

59. Documented in the *Geheimes Staatsarchiv Preussischer Kulturbesitz* (Secret State Archive, Prussian Cultural Possession), Mental Asylum Files Breslau, Vol. 12 (Berlin 1912), p. 123.

60. See note 10, MK 11288.

## 6. Breslau

1. Wilhelm II, "Der neue Name der Universität" (1910), in D. H. Klein, ed., *Breslau. Ein Lesebuch* (Husum 1988).

2. J. Raecke, "Alois Alzheimer," *Archiv für Psychiatrie und Nervenkrankheiten* 56 (1916): 1–6.

3. A. Kiejna, *Der Breslauer Zeitabschnitt von Alois Alzheimer und zur Eröffnung seines Geburtshauses als Gedenk- und Tagungsstätte*, Marktbreit, December 19, 1995 (unpublished).

4. K.-J. Neumärker, *Karl Bonhoeffer* (Leipzig 1990).

5. A. Alzheimer, "Über eine eigenartige Erkrankung des zentralen Nervensystems mit bulbären Symptomen und schmerzhaften spastischen Krampfzuständen der Extremitäten," *Zeitschrift für die Gesamte Neurologie und Psychiatrie* 33 (1916): 45–59 (posthumously edited by W. Spielmeyer).

6. Documented in Breslauer Psychiatrisch–Neurologische Vereinigung, meeting of February 17, 1913, in *Berliner Klinische Wochenschrift* 19 (1913): 1–8.

7. Franz Nissl, "Kleinere Mitteilungen zum Andenken an Alois Alzheimer," *Allgemeine Zeitschrift für Psychiatrie und Psychisch-Gerichtliche Medizin* 73 (1916): 96–107.

8. *Wiesbadener Bade-Blatt*, health resort lists of April 13, 1913, and May 23, 1913.

9. E. Kraepelin, *Lebenserinnerungen*, ed. H. Hippius, H. Peters, and H. Ploog (Berlin 1983), p. 172.

10. Documented in Secret State Archive, Prussian Cultural Possession, Files of the Breslau Mental Asylum, Vol. 5 (Berlin 1912), p. 27.

11. A. Alzheimer, "Fälle von Methylalkoholvergiftungen," *Deutsche Medizinische Wochenschrift* 41 (1915): 635.

12. A. Alzheimer, "Der Krieg und die Nerven," *Sonderdruck Breslau* (1915).

13. R. Gaupp, "Alois Alzheimer," *Münchner Medizinische Wochenschrift* 63 (1916): 195–196.

14. Letter from G. Stertz to R. Gaupp, December 12, 1915, Alois Alzheimer's birthplace, Marktbreit (unpublished).

15. *Schlesische Zeitung*, December 21, 1915.

16. See note 8.

17. C. Neisser, "Verhandlungen psychiatrischer Vereine. 101 Sitzung des

Ostdeutschen Vereins für Psychiatrie am 9 Dezember 1916," *Allgemeine Zeitschrift für Psychiatrie und Psychisch-Gerichtliche Medizin* 73 (1917): 369–372.

## 7. Alzheimer's: The Career of a Disease

1. A. Alzheimer, "Über eigenartige Krankheitsfälle des späteren Alters," *Zeitschrift für die Gesamte Neurologie und Psychiatrie* 4 (1911): 356–385.

2. G. R. Lafora, "Beitrag zur Kenntnis der Alzheimerschen Krankheit oder präsenilen Demenz mit Herdsymptomen," *Zeitschrift für die Gesamte Neurologie und Psychiatrie* 6 (1911): 15–20.

3. Franz Nissl, "Kleinere Mittelungen zum Andenken an Alois Alzheimer," in *Allgemeine Zeitschrift für Psychiatrie und Psychisch-Gerichtliche Medizin* 73 (1916): 96–107.

4. G. Stertz, "Das wissenschaftliche Wirken Alois Alzheimers," *Berliner Klinische Wochenschrift* 9 (1916): 235–238.

5. W. Spielmeyer, "Alzheimer's Lebenswerk," *Zeitschrift für die Gesamte Neurologie und Psychiatrie* 33 (1916): 1–41.

6. K. Kleist and K. Herz, "Die Alzheimerische Krankheit" *Programme der Medizinische Filmwoche V/188* (1925–1926).

7. G. Stertz, "Zu Fragen der Alzheimerischen Krankheit," *Allgemeine Zeitschrift für Psychiatrie und Psychisch-Gerichtliche Medizin* 37 (1921–1922): 336–339.

8. E. Grünthal, "Über die Alzheimerische Krankheit," *Zeitschrift für die Gesamte Neurologie und Psychiatrie* 101 (1926): 128–157.

9. E. Grünthal, "Klinisch-anatomisch vergleichende Untersuchungen über den Greisenblödsinn," *Zeitschrift für die Gesamte Neurologie und Psychiatrie* 111 (1927): 766–818.

10. J. Schottky, "Über praesenile Verblödungen," *Zeitschrift für die Gesamte Neurologie und Psychiatrie* 140 (1932): 333–397.

11. H. Pittrich, "Die Alzheimerische Krankheit," Reich Institute for Film and Image in Science and Teaching, University Film C 387/1941, Berlin 1941.

12. E. Albert, "Senile Demenz und Alzheimerische Krankheit als Ausdruck des gleichen Krankheitsgeschehens," *Fortschritte der Neurologie und Psychiatrie* 12 (1964): 625–672.

13. J. E. Meyer and H. Lauter, "Clinical and Nosological Concepts of Senile Dementia," in C. Mueller and L. Ciompi, eds., *Senile Dementia* (Stuttgart/Bern 1968), pp. 13–26.

14. E. Albert, "On the Nosology of Senile Dementia," in C. Mueller and L. Ciompi, eds., *Senile Dementia* (Stuttgart/Bern 1968), pp. 33–34.

15. J. A. N. Corsellis and P. H. Evans, "The Relation of Stenosis of the Extracranial Cerebral Arteries to Mental Disorder and Cerebral Degeneration in Old Age," *Proceedings of the International Congress of Neuropathology* 5 (1965): 546.

16. B. E. Tomlinson, G. Blessed, and M. Roth, "Observations on the Brains of Demented Old People," *Journal of Neurological Sciences* 11 (1970): 205–242.

17. V. C. Hachinski, N. A. Lassen, and J. Marshal, "Multiinfarct Dementia: A Cause of Mental Deterioration in the Elderly," *Lancet* 27 (1974): 207–209.

18. T. Klotz, K. Hurrelmann, and H. U. Eickenberg, "Der frühe Tod des starken Geschlechts," *Deutsches Ärtzeblatt* 95(9, February 27, 1998): 21.

19. *Apropos Rita Hayworth*, with an essay by Marli Feldvoss (Frankfurt 1996).

20. *Frankfurter Allgemeine Zeitung*, January 31, 1995.

21. Robert Katzman, "The Prevalence and Malignancy of Alzheimer's Disease: A Major Killer," *Archives of Neurology* 33 (1976).

22. "Alterskrankheit Alzheimer," *Der Spiegel* 25, June 19, 1989.

23. *Bildzeitung*, April 18, 1998.

# Glossary

Although the authors have made every effort to write in the most comprehensible language possible, in a book on a medical topic some specialized terms must be used, particularly in quotations. Because insertions and footnotes impede the flow of the text, these specialized terms are presented in this glossary.

AGORAPHOBIA: An irrational fear of leaving a familiar setting or venturing into open spaces, often associated with panic attacks.

AMAUROTIC IDIOCY: Lipometabolic disorder associated with visual disturbances, loss of intelligence, and paresis.

AMNESIA: Loss of memory.

APEX BEAT: Vibration of the anterior chest wall caused by the heartbeat.

ARTERIOSCLEROSIS: Thickening and loss of elasticity of the arterial walls, also known as hardening of the arteries.

ATHEROMATOUS DEGENERATION: Changes in the lining of the arteries caused by arteriosclerosis.

ATROPHY: Shrinkage (e.g., of the brain or other organ).

AUSCULTATION: Act of listening to sounds that come from within the body.

BINSWANGER'S DISEASE: Common form of a vascular dementia (strokelike, affecting the blood vessels of the brain).

CAPILLARIES, CAPILLARY VESSELS: The smallest blood vessels.

CATATONIA: Psychomotor disturbances characterized by alternating periods of physical rigidity, negativism, or stupor; may occur in schizophrenia, mood disorders, or organic mental disorders.

CONFABULATIONS: Illogical narratives or bizarre or tangential responses; stories a patient makes up to cover gaps in memory.

CREUTZFELDT–JAKOB DISEASE: Fatal disease of the central nervous system characterized by ataxia, abnormalities of gait and speech, and dementia. One of the *slow virus diseases*.

DEMENTIA: Loss of mental functions. If the loss appears before age sixty-five, it is called *presenile dementia*.

DEMENTIA PARALYTICA: Term for *general paresis*.

DEMENTIA PRAECOX: Term for *schizophrenia* that can be traced back to Emil Kraepelin.

DUCHENNE–ERB PARALYSIS (ERB PALSY): Paralysis of the nerves of the upper arm.

ECLAMPSIA: A severe toxic disturbance, usually during late pregnancy, characterized by hypertension, excessive weight gain, edema, and eventually convulsions and coma.

ENCEPHALITIS: Inflammation of the brain.

ENCEPHALOGRAPHY: Name for various obsolete methods of imaging brain activity. To depict the spatial relations in the brain, in *pneumencephalography* the brain is filled with air and X-rayed. Encephalography has been replaced by modern brain-scanning techniques.

ENDOGENOUS: Developed in the body. Endogenous diseases can be traced back to causes such as inherited predispositions, prenatal influences, or idiosyncratic physical traits.

ERB–CHARCOT DISEASE: A general paresis that begins during childhood, originates in the spinal cord, and is associated with spasticity in the legs.

ERB POINT: A stimulus point located approximately 7 centimeters above the clavicle with which the nerve network of the shoulder can be excited.

FIBRILS: Microscopically thin, spindly part of a nerve fiber.

GANGLIA: Nerve cells.

GENERAL PARESIS: Previously known as softening of the brain, refers to the late form of syphilis in which the syphilis pathogen penetrates the brain and causes clearly recognizable changes, particularly in the cerebral cortex; accompanying this are inflammation of the blood vessels and later degenerative processes of the nerve tissue, causing atrophy of the cerebral cortex. Also known as paretic neurosyphilis.

GLIA: The nervous system's supporting tissue located between the nerve cells, thought to have important metabolic functions. Also known as neuroglia.

GYRUS (pl., *gyri*): Rounded elevations visible on the surface of the brain.

HISTOPATHOLOGY: Science of viewing pathological changes of the body's tissue under the microscope.

HYSTERIA: Collective term for several psychosomatic disorders with variable physical and mental signs such as paralysis, fainting, and headaches, usually reflecting a psychological conflict or need.

LOGOCLONIA: Rhythmic repetition of the last syllable of a word.

LUES: Another name for *syphilis*.

MANIA: Emotional disorder characterized by an elevated mood and overactivity. (Hypomania is a mild form of mania.)

MENINGOMYELITIS: Inflammation of the brain and spinal cord.

MICROANGIOPATHY: Constricting disease of the wall of the capillaries that often occludes these vessels.

NEPHRITIS: Inflammation of the kidneys.

NEURASTHENIA: Fatigue or weakness of the nerves.

NEUROPATHOLOGY: Science of viewing changes in the brain under the microscope after death to detect diseases of the nervous system.

NOSOLOGY: Systematic description and classification of diseases.

PARANOIA: Mental disorder characterized by delusional ideas such as the idea that one is being persecuted.

PARAPHASIA: Mental disorder in which one loses the ability to speak intelligibly.

PATELLAR REFLEX: Knee tendon reflex.

PATHOLOGY: Science of diseases and their effects on the body.

PERCUSSION: Tapping on the surface of the body for diagnostic purposes.

PERSEVERATION: Uncontrollable repetition of a previously appropriate or correct response when the repeated response has become inappropriate or incorrect.

PLAQUES: Sharply demarcated lesions consisting of protein deposited between nerve cells in the brain in Alzheimer's disease.

POLLUTION: Obsolete term for spontaneous nocturnal ejaculation of semen, often associated with sexual dreams.

PRESBYOPHRENIA: Age-conditioned loss of mental abilities associated with severe amnesia, hyperactivity, euphoria, and disconnected narratives.

PSYCHOPATHY: Obsolete term for a predominantly inherited personality disorder.

PSYCHOSIS: Mental disorder in which the psychological functions are so impaired that connection to reality is lost or the ability to meet the usual demands of life is disturbed.

PULMONIC SOUND: The heart sound that can be heard over the pulmonary arteries.

PUPILLOPLEGIA: Immobility of the pupils, which can be conditioned by paralysis of the muscles that contract the pupils or by a deformity of the rim of the pupil but results primarily from a paralysis of the nerves that direct the pupils' movements. Failure of the pupils to contract in response to light can be an important indication of various brain diseases, including general paresis.

SALVARSAN: First cure for syphilis, an antibacterial arsenic-benzene combination.

SCHIZOPHRENIA: A name introduced by Eugen Bleuler for a form of psychosis characterized by both healthy and altered forms of experience and behavior; Emil Kraepelin called this disease *dementia praecox*.

SENILE: Very old; aged.

SENIUM PRAECOX: Premature aging.

SERODIAGNOSIS: Diagnosis of disease by analysis of blood serum.

SLOW VIRUS DISEASES: Insidious infectious diseases caused by viruses that emerge after a long period of incubation.

SUBCORTICAL: Located beneath the cerebral cortex.

SYPHILIS: Infectious disease (usually sexually transmitted), also called *lues*, that can attack the nervous system if left untreated.

TRAUMA: Injury and the damage associated with it. A psychological trauma can be caused by an especially strong mental shock and can lead to psychiatric or psychosomatic illnesses.

VIRGO INTACTA: Virgin; a female who has not had sexual intercourse.

# Internet Resources

Today, the Internet provides a wealth of information on Alzheimer's disease and its treatment as well as state-by-state services, support groups, and many other related topics. Here is a selection of groups and organizations, with their Web site addresses.

## Alzheimer's Association

The largest U.S. voluntary health organization supporting Alzheimer research and care, this association provides information on family caregivers, physicians and care professionals, and related topics (*see* www.alz.org).

## Alzheimer's Disease Educational Referral Center (ADEAR)
A Service of the National Institute on Aging

A division of the National Institutes of Health (NIH), ADEAR provides information on caregiving, research centers, clinical trials, and publications (*phone* 1-800-438-4380 or *see* www.alzheimers.org).

## Alzheimer's Disease International

This is the major umbrella organization of Alzheimer's associations around the world (*see* www.alz.co.uk).

## Alzheimer's Society (United Kingdom)
*See* www.alzheimers.org.uk.

## Alzheimer's Society of Canada
*See* www.alzheimer.ca.

## The Cognitive Neurology and Alzheimer's Disease Center (CN-ADC)
Northwestern University Medical School

CN-ADC provides information for caregivers, healthcare providers, investigators, and patients (*see* www.brain.neu.edu).

*MEDLINEplus*
A service of the U.S. National Library of Medicine and the National Institutes of Health

MEDLINE*plus* offers up-to-date medical news and information for patients or friends/parents of patients diagnosed with Alzheimer's disease (*see* www.nlm.nih.gov/medlineplus/alzheimersdisease.html).

*National Institutes of Health*
U.S. Department of Health and Human Services

Information here is available in both English and Spanish. Find out more about Alzheimer's disease by searching the NIH Web site (*see* www.nih.gov).

*Senior Resource*

This site offers information on a state-by-state basis in regard to housing, financial planning, and insurance pointers. To learn about programs and services available in your area, *see* seniorresource.com.

# Index

Page numbers for figures are followed by f. Initial articles (e.g., *The, Das*) are ignored in sorting. Numbers and dates are sorted as spelled. Names of institutions and book/article/film titles appear as cited in this text (English translation vs. original language).

Printed in the USA
CPSIA information can be obtained
at www.ICGtesting.com
JSHW021321221024
72173JS00011B/1625